a LANGE medical book

PRACTICE GUIDELINES In Primary Care 2002

Ralph Gonzales, MD, MSPH

Associate Professor
Division of General Internal Medicine
Department of Medicine
University of California, San Francisco
San Francisco, California

Jean S. Kutner, MD, MSPH

Assistant Professor
Division of General Internal Medicine
Department of Medicine
University of Colorado Health Sciences Center
Denver, Colorado

Lange Medical Books/McGraw-Hill
Medical Publishing Division

New York Chicago San Francisco Lisbon London
Madrid Mexico City Milan New Delhi San Juan
Seoul Singapore Sydney Tokyo Toronto

McGraw-Hill

*A Division of The **McGraw-Hill** Companies*

Practice Guidelines in Primary Care 2002

1 2 3 4 5 6 7 8 9 0 WBC/WBC 0 9 8 7 6 5 4 3 2

ISBN 0-07-137797-2
ISSN 1528-1612

Notice

Medicine is an ever-changing science. As new research and clinical experience broaden our knowledge, changes in treatment and drug therapy are required. The authors and the publisher of this work have checked with sources believed to be reliable in their efforts to provide information that is complete and generally in accord with the standards accepted at the time of publication. However, in view of the possibility of human error or changes in medical sciences, neither the authors nor the publisher nor any other party who has been involved in the preparation or publication of this work warrants that the information contained herein is in every respect accurate or complete, and they disclaim all responsibility for any errors or ommissions or for the results obtained from use of the information contained in this work. Readers are encouraged to confirm the information contained herein with other sources. For example and in particular, readers are advised to check the product information sheet included in the package of each drug they plan to administer to be certain that the information contained in this work is accurate and that changes have not been made in the recommended dose or in the contraindications for administration. This recommendation is of particular importance in connection with new or infrequently used drugs.

This book was set by International Typesetting and Composition.

Webcom Limited was printer and binder.

Contents

DISEASE SCREENING

DISEASE PREVENTION

DISEASE MANAGEMENT

APPENDICES

Preface

PURPOSE

Now annually updated, *Practice Guidelines in Primary Care 2002* is intended for primary care clinicians. These include not only residents and practicing physicians in the specialties of family medicine, internal medicine, pediatrics, and obstetrics and gynecology, but also medical and nursing students during their ambulatory care rotations, registered nurses, nurse practitioners, and physician's assistants. Its purpose is to make screening and primary prevention and treatment recommendations readily accessible and available for clinical decision making.

These types of recommendations are issued regularly by governmental agencies, expert panels, medical specialty organizations, and other professional and scientific organizations. *Practice Guidelines in Primary Care 2002* is essential for the busy clinician. Guidelines are continually being published by organizations that express different positions on the same topics, and current guidelines require revision as new evidence from clinical and outcomes research emerges. The intent of this guide is to help clinicians select the most appropriate clinical preventive services and interventions for a given situation.

CONTENT

A major focus of *Practice Guidelines in Primary Care 2002* is screening and primary prevention, both of which apply only to persons without evidence of current disease. **Screening** encompasses tests or examinations intended to identify persons who require specific interventions. **Primary prevention** describes interventions intended to prevent the onset of particular conditions.

An effective screening test is one that detects a condition earlier than would be detected without screening and has sufficient accuracy to avoid producing large numbers of false-positive or false-negative results. Screening is appropriate only if this early detection improves health outcomes. To be considered effective, preventive interventions should decrease disease-specific morbidity or mortality.

Beginning with this edition, *Practice Guidelines in Primary Care* will be annually updated to keep pace with ongoing changes in clinical practice guidelines. For this new edition, we have greatly expanded the section that provides disease management algorithms for the most common conditions managed by primary care clinicians. In addition, we have included useful screening instruments.

A list of the organizations that have developed guidelines included in *Practice Guidelines in Primary Care 2002*, along with their current Internet addresses, is located in the Appendix.

ACKNOWLEDGMENT

We are grateful to Lisa Scatena, MD for her valuable assistance in researching and preparing this new edition of *Practice Guidelines in Primary Care*.

Ralph Gonzales, MD, MSPH
Jean S. Kutner, MD, MSPH

San Francisco, California
Denver, Colorado
January 2002

1
Disease Screening

ALCOHOL ABUSE & DEPENDENCE

Disease Screening	Organization	Date	Population	Recommendations	Comments	Source
Alcohol Abuse & Dependence	GAPS AAP Bright Futures	1997 1995	Adolescents	Ask all adolescents annually about their use of alcohol. Parents should also routinely receive instructions on monitoring their adolescent's social and recreational activities for use of alcohol.[a]	The finding of alcohol use or abuse should provoke an assessment of other conditions that co-vary with alcohol abuse, such as cigarette smoking, sexual activity, and mood disorders. Guidelines on treatment of alcohol abuse in adolescence have been published. (J Am Acad Child Adolesc Psychiatry 1998;37:122)	Arch Pediatr Adolesc Med 1997;151:123 Pediatrics 1995;95:439
	USPSTF CTF	1996 1994	Adolescents and adults	Screen all adolescents and adults using relevant history or a standardized screening instrument (see Appendix I for CAGE and AUDIT instruments).	A recent systematic review concluded that the Alcohol Use Disorders Identification Test (AUDIT) was most effective in identifying subjects with at-risk, hazardous, or harmful drinking (sensitivity, 51%–79%; specificity, 78%–96%); while the CAGE questions proved superior for detecting alcohol abuse and dependence (sensitivity, 43%–94%; specificity 70%–97%). (Arch Intern Med 2000;160:1977) Screening coupled with brief physician advice is cost-effective (5.6:1). (Med Care 2000;38:7)	

ALCOHOL ABUSE & DEPENDENCE

Disease Screening	Organization	Date	Population	Recommendations	Comments	Source
Alcohol Abuse & Dependence (continued)	ACOG AAP	1997	Pregnant women	Counsel all pregnant women regarding the maternal health and fetal effects of alcohol during pregnancy.		AAP and ACOG: Guidelines for Perinatal Care, 4th ed. ACOG, 1997.

[a]The AAP also acknowledges the importance of family attitudes toward alcohol and recommends that clinicians urge parents to use alcohol safely and in moderation, to restrict children from family alcohol supplies, and to recognize the influence their own drinking patterns can have on their children and parenting.

ANEMIA

Disease Screening	Organization	Date	Population	Recommendations	Comments	Source
Anemia, Iron-Deficient	AAP	1993	Neonates	Universal hematocrit screening is not recommended.		Pediatrics 1993;92:474
	USPSTF	1996	Infants ages 6–12 months	Perform selective, single hemoglobin or hematocrit screening for high-risk infants.[a]		
	USPSTF	1996	Pregnant women	Screen all women with hemoglobin or hematocrit at first prenatal visit.	When acute stress or inflammatory disorders are not present, a serum ferritin level is the most accurate test for evaluating iron deficiency anemia. Among women of childbearing age, a cut-off of 15 mg/dL has sensitivity of 75%, specificity of 98%. (Br J Haematol 1993;85:787)	

[a]Includes infants living in poverty, blacks, Native Americans and Alaska Natives, immigrants from developing countries, preterm and low birthweight infants, and infants whose principal dietary intake is unfortified cow's milk.

CANCER, BLADDER

Disease Screening	Organization	Date	Population	Recommendations	Comments	Source
Cancer, Bladder	AAFP USPSTF CTF	2000 1996 1994	Asymptomatic persons[a]	Routine screening with microscopic urinalysis, urine dipstick, or urine cytology is not recommended.	Positive predictive value of serial dipstick screening for malignancy: 68% (USPSTF). Dipstick testing is sensitive and specific for hematuria, but hematuria is not specific for bladder cancer.	www.aafp.org/exam/negative.html

[a]Increased risk: exposure to azodyes, aromatic amines, and 4-aminobiphenyl; employment in the leather, tire, or rubber industries; and cigarette smoking (OR/RR 1.5–7.0). Persons working in high-risk professions may be eligible for screening at the worksite, although the benefit of this has not been determined. People who smoke should be advised that smoking significantly increases the risk for bladder cancer, and all smokers should be routinely counseled to quit smoking. A high index of suspicion should be maintained in anyone with a history of smoking or exposure to another risk factor. (USPSTF)

CANCER, BREAST

Disease Screening	Organization	Date	Population[a]	Recommendations	Comments	Source
Cancer, Breast	ACS	2000	Women age > 20 years	Monthly breast self exam (BSE)	The value of BSE in reducing breast cancer mortality remains unproved. (Br J Cancer 1993;68:208) BSE is considered supplemental to, rather than a substitute for, screening by CBE and mammography.	www3.cancer/org/ cancerinfo
	ACS ACOG	2000	Women ages 20–39 years	Clinician breast examination (CBE) every 3 years		www3.cancer.org/ cancerinfo www.acog.org
	ACS ACOG	2000 1996	Women age ≥ 40 years	Mammography and CBE yearly	The CBE should be conducted close in time to the scheduled mammogram.	www3.cancer.org/ cancerinfo www.acog.org
	NCI AMA	2001 1989	Women ages 40–49 years	Mammography every 1–2 years and CBE yearly	Screening mammography initiated between the ages of 40 and 49 reduces breast cancer mortality, an effect that can be identified 10–12 years after the start of screening. A portion of this benefit may be due to mammography performed after age 49.	http://cancernet. nci.nih.gov JAMA 1989;261(17): 2535

CANCER, BREAST

Disease Screening	Organization	Date	Population[a]	Recommendations	Comments	Source
Cancer, Breast (continued)	NIH AAFP	1997	Women ages 40–49 years	Counsel about risks/benefits of mammography and CBE.	Extending screening to include ages 40–49 improves life expectancy by 2.5 days at a cost of $676/woman. Incremental cost-effectiveness is $105,000 per year of life saved. (Ann Intern Med 1997;127:955) RCTs consistently demonstrate no benefit from screening in the first 5–7 years after study entry. At 10–12 years, benefit is uncertain. (J Natl Cancer Inst 1993;85(20):1644) Number needed to screen to save 1 life = 2500. (J Natl Cancer Inst 1997;89(14):1015) Thirty percent of all women screened annually at ages 40–49 will have at least 1 false-positive mammogram. (J Natl Cancer Inst 1997;22:139) Risk-based recommendations may assist in counseling. (J Clin Oncol 1998;16(9):3105)	NIH Consensus Statement 1997;15(1):1 J Natl Cancer Inst 1997;89(14):1015 www.aafp.org/exam?pos_gen_sta.html

Disease Screening	Organization	Date	Population[a]	Recommendations	Comments	Source
Cancer, Breast (continued)	NCI CTF ACP AMA	2001 1994 1991 1989	Women ages 50–69 years	Mammography and CBE yearly	For women ages 50–69, all studies show mortality reductions with screening of about 30% at 10–12 years. (J Natl Cancer Inst 1993;85(20):1644) Screening women ages 50–69 years improves life expectancy by 12 days at a cost of $704/woman, with a cost-effectiveness ratio of $21,400 per year of life saved. (Ann Intern Med 1997;127:955)	http://cancernet.nci.nih.gov/ JAMA 1989;261(17):2535 Common Screening Tests. ACP, 1991.
	AAFP ACPM USPSTF	2000 1996 1996	Women ages 50–69 years	Mammography and CBE every 1–2 years		www.aafp.org/exam/pos_gen_sta.html www.acpm.org/breast.htm
	NCI	2001	Women age ≥ 70 years	Screening may or may not be helpful		http://cancernet.nci.nih.gov

CANCER, BREAST

Disease Screening	Organization	Date	Population[a]	Recommendations	Comments	Source
Cancer, Breast (continued)	ACPM USPSTF AGS	1996 1996 1989	Women age ≥ 70 years	Mammography and CBE every 1–2 years AGS recommends, in addition, monthly BSE.	Currently available data for women age > 70 are inadequate to judge the effectiveness of screening. (J Natl Cancer Inst 1993;85(20):1644)	www.acpm.org/breast.htm J Am Geriatr Soc 1989;37(9):883

[a]Women with a mother and sister with breast cancer have an RR > 4.0 of developing breast cancer. It is likely that < 10% of all breast cancer in western countries is attributable to genetic predisposition. It has been estimated that 25% of breast cancers diagnosed before age 40 years are attributable to *BRCA1* mutations. Studies have not addressed when to begin breast cancer screening, and at what intervals, for women at high risk of breast cancer because of genetic predisposition. (Annu Rev Public Health 1996;17:47)

CANCER, CERVICAL

Disease Screening	Organization	Date	Population	Recommendations[a]	Comments	Source
Cancer, Cervical	NCI ACS ACOG GAPS Bright Futures	2001 2000 1998 1994 1994	Women who are or have been sexually active Or Women age > 18 years[b]	Pap smear (with endocervical brush and spatula) and pelvic exam every year; if > 3 consecutive normal exams, may perform less frequently at physician discretion	Lead time from precancerous lesions to invasive cancer is 8–9 years. (Clinician's Handbook of Preventive Services. US Government Printing Office, 1994) Single screening Pap test for detecting CIN grades I and II has sensitivity 14–99%, specificity 24–96%. (Am J Epidemiol 1995; 141:680) The rate of false-negative results may be as high as 50%. An estimated 1/2 to 2/3 of false-negative results are caused by inadequate specimen collection and by misinterpreting or not observing abnormal cells. Recent studies have provided strong evidence that HPV DNA testing may have a strong role in identifying precancerous lesions and managing minor Pap abnormalities. (Ann Intern Med 2000;133:1021–1024). 20–60% reduction in cervical cancer mortality rates after implementation of screening programs. (Ann Intern Med 1990;113(3):214)	http://www3.cancer/org/cancerinfo http://cancernet.nci.nih.giv/ http://www.acog.org Can Med Assoc J 1991;144:313

CANCER, CERVICAL

Disease Screening	Organization	Date	Population	Recommendations[a]	Comments	Source
Cancer, Cervical (continued)	AAFP USPSTF ACP	2000 1996 1990	Women who have ever had sex and have a cervix[b]	Pap smear at least every 3 years		www.aafp.org/exam/pos_gen_sta.html Ann Intern Med 1990;113(3):214
	ACPM CTF	1996 1994	Women who have ever had sex[b]	Pap smear every year for 2 years; if 2 normal annual smears, lengthen screening interval to 3 years at physician discretion		www.acpm.org/cervical.htm
	ACPM USPSTF	1996 1996	Women age > 65 years	Discontinue screening if: regular screening, 2 satisfactory smears, and no abnormal smears within previous 9 years. If no previous screening, 3 normal smears before discontinuation	28–64% of women age > 65 have never had a Pap smear or have not had one done within 3 years. (Mt Sinai J Med 1985;52:284) In one study, women 65 years of age and older were 21% less likely than younger women to ever have had a Pap test and 33% less likely to have had a Pap test recently. Physician recommendation is the strongest predictor of whether a woman receives a Pap test. (Ann Intern Med 2000;133:1021–1024)	www.acpm.org/cervical.htm

Disease Screening	Organization	Date	Population	Recommendations[a]	Comments	Source
Cancer, Cervical (continued)	AGS CTF	2000 1994	Women age > 65 years	Pap smear every 1–3 years until age 70. If no or insufficient prior Pap smears, 2 annual smears before discontinuation.	Cervical cancer is causally related to infection with HPV. (http://odp.od.nih.gov/consensus/) Beyond age 70, there is little evidence for or against screening women who have been regularly screened in previous years. Individual circumstances such as the patient's life expectancy, ability to undergo treatment if cancer is detected, and ability to cooperate with and tolerate the Pap smear procedure may obviate the need for cervical cancer screening.	http://www.americangeriatrics.org/products/positionpapers/cer_carc_2000.shtml

[a]Risk factors for cervical cancer: sexual activity, early onset of sexual intercourse, history of multiple sexual partners or male sexual partners who have had multiple partners, male partners whose other sexual partners have had cervical cancer, history of STDs (especially HPV, HIV, HSV), immunosuppression, smoking, history of cervical dysplasia or endometrial, vaginal, or vulvar cancer, and no previous screening (may indicate more frequent screening interval). (Ann Intern Med 2000;133:1021–1024) ((http://www.cancernet.nci.nih.gov/clinpdq/screening); Ann Intern Med 1990;113(3):214)

[b]If sexual history is unknown or considered unreliable, screening should begin at age 18 years.

Disease Screening	Organization	Date	Population	Recommendations	Comments	Source
Cancer, Colorectal	ASCRS	1999	Age ≥ 50 years, low or average risk[b]	Yearly DRE and one of the following: FOBT[a] and flexible sigmoidoscopy every 5 years OR Total colon exam (colonscopy or double contrast barium enema and proctosigmoidoscopy)	Beginning in July 2001, Medicare will cover screening colonoscopy every 10 years for people who are NOT at high risk for colon cancer. (HCFA Press Release, 3/14/01; www.hcfa.gov)	www.fascrs.org/

CANCER, COLORECTAL

Disease Screening	Organization	Date	Population	Recommendations	Comments	Source
Cancer, Colorectal (continued)	NCI	2001	Ages 50–80 years	Guaiac-based FOBT every 1–2 years Regular screening by flexible sigmoidoscopy may decrease mortality from colon cancer. There is insufficient evidence to determine optimal interval.	Models indicate that screening persons > 50 years for colorectal cancer with annual FOBT, flexible sigmoidoscopy, or a single colonoscopy compares favorably with screening mammography in women age > 50 years in the cost per year of life saved. (N Engl J Med 1995;332(13):861) Screening for colorectal cancer, even in the setting of imperfect compliance, significantly reduces colorectal cancer mortality at costs comparable to other cancer screening procedures. (JAMA 2000;284:1954–1961) Low compliance rates may render colonoscopy every 10 years the most cost-effective primary screening strategy for colorectal cancer. (Ann Intern Med 2000;133:573–584) The use of either annual or biennial FOBT reduces the incidence of colorectal cancer (incidence ratios 0.80 for annual and 0.83 for biennial screening). (N Engl J Med 2000;343:1603) US military veterans who did not have colorectal cancer were 50% more likely to have had endoscopic procedures. (Ann Intern Med 1995;123:904)	http://cancernet.nci.nih.gov/

CANCER, COLORECTAL

Disease Screening	Organization	Date	Population	Recommendations	Comments	Source
Cancer, Colorectal (continued)	ACS AGA	2000 1997	Age ≥ 50 years[b]	Yearly FOBT + flexible sigmoidoscopy and DRE every 5 years[a] OR Colonoscopy + DRE every 10 years OR Double contrast BE + DRE every 5–10 years		http://www3.cancer.org/cancerinfo http://www.gastrojournal.org/cgi/reprint/112/2/594.pdf (Gastroenterology 1997;112:594–642)
	AAFP	2000	Age > 50 years	Yearly FOBT, flexible sigmoidoscopy, colonoscopy, or barium enema.		http://www.aafp.org/exam/pos_gen_guide.html
	ACP	1997	Ages 50–70 years	Yearly FOBT[a] and flexible sigmoidoscopy, colonoscopy, or air contrast BE every 10 years		www.acponline.org/journals/annals/15may97/ppcolo1.htm
	USPSTF	1996	Age > 50 years[b]	Yearly FOBT OR Flexible sigmoidoscopy (no periodicity), or both There is insufficient evidence to recommend for or against DRE, BE, or colonoscopy.		

CANCER, COLORECTAL

[a]A positive result on an FOBT should be followed by a complete colorectal exam by colonoscopy. An alternative is flexible sigmoidoscopy and air-contrast BE. (Ann Intern Med 1997;126(10):808)

[b]Risk factors indicating need for earlier/more frequent screening: personal history of colorectal cancer or adenomatous polyps, colorectal cancer or polyps in a first-degree relative < 60 years old or in a second-degree relative of any age, personal history of chronic inflammatory bowel disease, and family with hereditary colorectal cancer syndromes. (Ann Intern Med 1998;128(1):900, N Engl J Med 1994;331(25):1669, N Engl J Med 1995;332(13):861) If history of colorectal cancer in first-degree relative, age 55 or younger, or 2 or more first-degree relatives of any ages, colonoscopy is recommended at age 40 or 10 years before the youngest case in the family, whichever is earlier. (http://www.fascrs.org)

CANCER, ENDOMETRIAL

Disease Screening	Organization	Date	Population	Recommendations	Comments	Source
Cancer, Endometrial	NCI	2000	All women	Routine screening of women for endometrial cancer is not recommended. There is insufficient evidence to establish whether a decrease in mortality from endometrial cancer occurs with screening by endometrial sampling or transvaginal ultrasound.	Presence of endometrial cells in Pap test from postmenopausal woman not taking exogenous hormones is abnormal and requires further evaluation. Endometrial thickness of < 4 mm on transvaginal ultrasound is associated with low risk of endometrial cancer. (Obstet Gynecol 1991;78(2):195)	http://cancernet.nci.nih.gov/
	ACS	2000	All women at high risk for endometrial cancer.[a]	Women at high risk for cancer of the uterus should have a sample of endometrial tissue examined when menopause begins.		http://www3.cancer.org/cancerinfo

[a]Increased endometrial cancer risk: history of infertility, obesity, previous abnormal uterine bleeding, estrogen therapy unopposed by progestin intake, tamoxifen therapy, and genetic mutations associated with hereditary nonpolyposis colon cancer. (Obstet Gynecol 1999;93(4):594, http://cancernet.nci.nih.gov/pdq.html)

CANCER, GASTRIC

Disease Screening	Organization	Date	Population	Recommendations	Comments	Source
Cancer, Gastric	NCI	2000	Adults in United States	Routine screening of the US population is not recommended. There is insufficient evidence to establish that screening would result in a decrease in mortality from gastric cancer in the US population.	Studies of screening in Japan (via barium x-ray) have demonstrated decreases in mortality in screened versus unscreened patients. (Int J Cancer 1995;60:45)	http://cancernet.nci.nih.gov/

CANCER, LIVER

Disease Screening	Organization	Date	Population	Recommendations	Comments	Source
Cancer, Liver (Hepatocellular Carcinoma)	Workshop on Screening for Hepatocellular Cancer (Indian Health Service, Fox Chase Cancer Center, CDC)	1989	High-risk children and adults[a]	HBsAg-positive carriers: α-fetoprotein level at least annually, preferably twice a year HBsAg-positive carriers with cirrhosis or family history of HCC: periodic ultrasound and α-fetoprotein HBsAg negative with cirrhosis or chronic liver disease: no screening recommendations		J Natl Cancer Inst 1991;83:916 MMWR 1990;39:619

[a]The incidence of HCC is high in persons positive for HBsAg for > 6 months. Especially high risk: males, cirrhosis, age > 45 years, and family history of HCC. (J Natl Cancer Inst 1991;83:916, Arch Intern Med 1989;149:1741)

CANCER, LUNG

Disease Screening	Organization	Date	Population	Recommendations	Comments	Source
Cancer, Lung	NCI AAFP ACS USPSTF CTF ACP ATS ACR	2001 2000 2000 1996 1994 1991 1983 1982	Asymptomatic persons	Routine screening for lung cancer with chest radiography or sputum cytology is not recommended.	All patients should be counseled against tobacco use. No significant benefit in terms of lung cancer mortality by screening with chest radiography and sputum cytology. (J Occup Med 1986;28:746) Annual low-dose chest CT in high-risk patients appears to increase detection of resectable cancer. Impact of screening on mortality has not been determined. (Lancet 1999;354(9173):99) Although there is public and political pressure, based on low-dose CT prevalence-screening data, to change clinical practice and to offer mass lung-cancer screening, there should be no compromise or shortcuts in the rigorous scientific process required to determine whether this process is justified. Well-designed studies should be conducted, completed, analyzed, and validated before a mass screening program is implemented. (N Engl J Med 2000;343:1627) (JAMA 2000;284:1980)	http://cancernet.nci.nih.gov/ http://www.aafp.org/exam/negative.html http://www3.cancer.org/cancerinfo Common Screening Tests. ACP, 1991. Am Rev Respir Dis 1984;130:565 www.acr.org

CANCER, ORAL

Disease Screening	Organization	Date	Population	Recommendations	Comments	Source
Cancer, Oral	NCI USPSTF CTF	2000 1996 1994	Asymptomatic persons	There is insufficient evidence to establish that screening would result in a decrease in mortality from oral cancer.		http://cancernet.nci.nih.gov/
	NIDR	1994	Asymptomatic persons	Screen during routine dental exam.		Detecting Oral Cancer: A Guide for Dentists. NIDR, 1994.
	USPSTF CTF	1996 1994	High-risk persons[a]	Consider annual oral exam.[b]		
	ACS	2000	Ages 20–40 years	Screen with oral exam (inspection and palpation of oral cavity) every 3 years.		http://www.cancer.org/guide/guidchec.html
	ACS	2000	Age > 40 years	Screen with annual oral exam.		http://www.cancer.org/guide/guidchec.html
	AGS	1991	Age > 60 years	Screen with annual oral exam.		J Am Geriatr Soc 1991;39(9):920

[a]Risk factors: regular alcohol or tobacco use.

[b]Inquire about alcohol and tobacco use and counsel about risk.

CANCER, OVARIAN

Disease Screening	Organization	Date	Population	Recommendations	Comments	Source
Cancer, Ovarian	NCI AAFP ACPM USPSTF ACP CTF	2000 2000 1997 1996 1994 1994	Asymptomatic women[a]	There is insufficient evidence to establish that screening for ovarian cancer with serum markers such as CA-125 levels, transvaginal ultrasound, or pelvic examinations would result in a decrease in mortality from ovarian cancer.	In asymptomatic women, pelvic exam has unknown sensitivity and specificity; abdominal ultrasound has specificity 97.7%, sensitivity 100%, positive predictive value 2.6%; transvaginal ultrasound has specificity 98.1%, sensitivity 100%, positive predictive value 22%; CA-125 has sensitivity 50% for stages I and II and 90% for stages III and IV, and specificity 97.6%, when followed by abdominal ultrasound. (Ann Intern Med 1993;118(11):838, http://www.acpm.org/ovary.htm)	http://www.cancernet.nci.nih.gov/ www.acpm.org/ovary.htm www.aafp.org/exam/negative.html Ann Intern Med 1994;121(2):124
	NIH	1994	Asymptomatic women[a]	Comprehensive family history and annual rectovaginal pelvic exam		NIH Consensus Statement 1994;12(3):1

CANCER, OVARIAN

[a]Risk factors: age > 60 years; low parity; personal history of endometrial, colon, or breast cancer; family history of ovarian cancer; and hereditary ovarian cancer syndrome. Lifetime risk of ovarian cancer in a woman with no affected relatives is 1 in 70. If 1 first-degree relative has ovarian cancer, lifetime risk is 5%. If 2 or more first-degree relatives have ovarian cancer, lifetime risk is 7%. Women with 2 or more family members affected by ovarian cancer have a 3% chance of having a hereditary ovarian cancer syndrome. These women have a 40% lifetime risk of ovarian cancer. There are no data demonstrating that screening high-risk women reduces their mortality from ovarian cancer. A low annual incidence (13.8/100,000) means that many people must be screened to find only a few cases of disease. (NIH Consensus Statement 1994;12(3):1, Ann Intern Med 1993;118(11):838)

Several large-scale studies designed to establish the effectiveness of general population screening for ovarian cancer have begun. Each uses transvaginal ultrasonography or a multimodal strategy in which elevated serum levels of CA-125 tumor marker prompt secondary testing with transvaginal ultrasonography. (Ann Intern Med 2000;133:1021–24)

CANCER, PANCREATIC

Disease Screening	Organization	Date	Population	Recommendations	Comments	Source
Cancer, Pancreatic	USPSTF CTF	1996 1994	Asymptomatic persons	Routine screening using abdominal palpation, ultrasonography, or serologic markers is not recommended.	Cigarette smoking has consistently been associated with increased risk of pancreatic cancer.	

Disease Screening	Organization	Date	Population	Recommendations	Comments	Source
Cancer, Prostate	NCI	2000	Asymptomatic men	Insufficient evidence to establish whether a decrease in mortality from prostate cancer occurs with screening by DRE, TRUS, or serum markers including PSA		http://cancernet.nci.nih.gov/
	ACS AUA	2000 2000	Men age ≥ 50 years[a]	Offer annual PSA and DRE if > 10-year life expectancy.[b]	DRE has sensitivity 50%, specificity 94%; PSA has sensitivity 67%, specificity 84%; TRUS has sensitivity 81%, specificity 84%. (JAMA 1994;272(10):773)	http://www3.cancer.org/cancerinfo Oncology 2000;14:267–286
	AAFP	2000	Men age 50–65 years	Counsel regarding the known risks and uncertain benefits of screening for prostate cancer.		http://www.aafp.org/exam/pos_gen_guide.html
	ACPM ACP	1998 1997	Men age > 50 years[a]	Describe potential benefits and known harms of screening with PSA and DRE, diagnosis, and treatment; listen to the patient's concerns; and individualize the decision to screen.	Data are not yet available to quantify the risks and benefits of screening for prostate cancer or to prove that treating clinically localized cancer reduces disease-specific mortality rates. (Ann Intern Med 1997;126(6):468)	www.acpm.org/prostate.htm Ann Intern Med 1997;126(6):480

CANCER, PROSTATE

Disease Screening	Organization	Date	Population	Recommendations	Comments	Source
Cancer, Prostate (continued)	USPSTF	1996	Men age > 50 years[a]	Routine screening with DRE, PSA, or TRUS is not recommended.		
	CTF	1994	Men age > 50 years[a]	Poor evidence to include or exclude DRE, insufficient evidence to include PSA, and fair evidence to exclude TRUS		

[a]Men in high-risk groups (2 or more affected first-degree relatives, blacks) should begin screening at a younger age (eg, 45 years). More data on the precise age to start prostate cancer screening are needed for men at high risk. No direct or indirect evidence quantifies the yield and predictive value of early detection efforts in higher-risk men. (http://www.cancer.org/guide/guidchec.html, http://auanet.org/pub_pat/policies/uroservices.html, Ann Intern Med 1997;126(6):480)

[b]Some elevations in PSA may be due to benign conditions of the prostate. The DRE should be performed by health care workers skilled in recognizing subtle prostate abnormalities, including those of symmetry and consistency, as well as the more classic findings of marked induration or nodules. DRE is less effective in detecting prostate carcinoma than is PSA. (http://www.cancer.org/guide/guidchec.html, http://auanet.org/pub_pat/policies/uroservices.html)

CANCER, SKIN

Disease Screening	Organization	Date	Population	Recommendations	Comments	Source
Cancer, Skin	NCI USPSTF CTF	2000 1996 1994	Asymptomatic persons	Insufficient evidence to establish whether a decrease in mortality occurs with routine examination of the skin. Insufficient evidence to recommend for or against routine screening using total-body skin exam.[a] Insufficient evidence to recommend for or against counseling patients to perform periodic skin self-exam.[b]		http://cancernet.nci.nih.gov/
	NIH AAD	1992 1992	Asymptomatic persons	Annual screening using total-body skin exam.		JAMA 1992;268(10):1314 J Am Acad Dermatol 1992;26:629
	ACPM	1998	Asymptomatic persons	Periodic total cutaneous examinations, targeting populations at high risk for malignant melanoma.[b] Insufficient evidence to characterize periodicity of skin examinations more precisely.		http://www.acpm.org/skincanc.htm

CANCER, SKIN

Disease Screening	Organization	Date	Population	Recommendations	Comments	Source
Cancer, Skin (continued)	ACS	2000	Ages 20–39 years	Screening with skin exam every 3 years		http://www3.cancer.org/cancerinfo
	ACS	2000	Age ≥ 40 years	Annual screening with skin exam		http://www3.cancer.org/cancerinfo

[a]Clinicians should remain alert for skin lesions with malignant features when examining patients for other reasons, particularly patients with established risk factors. Risk factors for skin cancer include: evidence of melanocytic precursors, large numbers of common moles, immunosuppression, family or personal history of skin cancer, substantial cumulative lifetime sun exposure, intermittent intense sun exposure or severe sunburns in childhood, freckles, poor tanning ability, and light skin, hair, and eye color. Appropriate biopsy specimens should be taken of suspicious lesions. Persons with melanocytic precursor or marker lesions are at substantially increased risk for malignant melanoma and should be referred to skin cancer specialists for evaluation and surveillance. (USPSTF)

[b]Consider educating patients with established risk factors for skin cancer (see above) concerning signs and symptoms suggesting skin cancer and the possible benefits of periodic self-exam. (USPSTF)

CANCER, TESTICULAR

Disease Screening	Organization	Date	Population	Recommendations	Comments	Source
Cancer, Testicular	NCI USPSTF CTF	2000 1996 1994	Asymptomatic men[a]	Insufficient evidence to recommend for or against routine screening by physician exam, patient self-exam, or tumor markers (α-fetoprotein, human chorionic gonadotropin). Insufficient evidence to establish that screening would result in a decrease in mortality from testicular cancer.		http://cancernet.nci.nih.gov/

[a]Patients with history of cryptorchidism, orchiopexy, or testicular atrophy should be informed of their increased risk for developing testicular cancer and counseled about screening. Such patients may then elect to be screened or to perform testicular self-exam. Adolescent and young adult males should be advised to seek prompt medical attention if they notice a scrotal abnormality. (USPSTF)

CANCER, THYROID

Disease Screening	Organization	Date	Population	Recommendations	Comments	Source
Cancer, Thyroid	AAFP USPSTF CTF	2000 1996 1994	Asymptomatic persons	Screening asymptomatic adults or children using either neck palpation or ultrasonography is not recommended.[a]	Neck palpation for nodules in asymptomatic individuals has sensitivity 15–38%; specificity 93–100%. Only a small proportion of nodular thyroid glands are neoplastic, resulting in a high false-positive rate. (USPSTF)	www.aafp.org/exam/negative.html

[a]Includes asymptomatic persons with a history of external upper-body irradiation in infancy or childhood.

CAROTID ARTERY STENOSIS

Disease Screening	Organization	Date	Population	Recommendations	Comments	Source
Carotid Artery Stenosis (asymptomatic)	AHA	1998	Ages 40–79 years	Screen asymptomatic patients (? interval) with < 5% surgical risk and > 5-year life expectancy.[a]	In the Asymptomatic Carotid Atherosclerosis Study, the actuarial 5-year risk of ipsilateral stroke, operative stroke, and death was ≅ 5% with CEA vs 11% in the control group. Combined surgical morbidity and mortality was 2.3%. (JAMA 1995;273:1421)	http://circ.ahajournals.org/cgi/content/full/97/5/501
	CNS	1997	Ages 40–79 years	Insufficient evidence to screen asymptomatic individuals because CEA recommendation is "uncertain" for > 60% stenosis.[b]		Can Med Assoc J 1997;157:653
	USPSTF	1996	Age > 60 years	Selective screening[c]		
	CTF	1994		Insufficient evidence to screen		
	SVS	1992		Selective screening[d]		J Vasc Surg 1992;15:469

CAROTID ARTERY STENOSIS

[a]If surgical risk is < 3% and life expectancy is > 5 years, ipsilateral CEA is acceptable for > 60% stenosis; if surgical risk is 35%, ipsilateral CEA is acceptable (but not proved) for > 75% bilateral stenoses.

[b]Recommend stenosis be documented with angiography using the method of the North American Symptomatic Carotid Endarterectomy Trial.

[c]Selective screening may be appropriate in the presence of other stroke risk factors, no contraindications to major surgery, and access to surgeons and centers with < 3% perioperative morbidity and mortality.

[d]Screen patients with audible carotid bruit, multiple risk factors for CAS, or those who are preparing for operation in another vascular bed using duplex scan. Recommend CEA for patients with > 75% stenosis with life expectancy > 5 years and surgical risk < 3%. Other candidates for CEA include those with CT scan evidence of silent embolization, mixed plaque consistency, or evidence that the lesion has progressed over 6 months.

CHILD ABUSE & NEGLECT

Disease Screening	Organization	Date	Population	Recommendations	Comments	Source
Child Abuse & Neglect	GAPS	1997	Children and adolescents	All teens should be asked annually about a history of emotional, physical, and sexual abuse.	By law, child abuse must be reported to appropriate authorities in all 50 states.	Arch Pediatr Adolesc Med 1997;151:123

CHOLESTEROL & LIPID DISORDERS, CHILDREN

Disease Screening	Organization	Date	Population	Recommendations	Comments	Source
Cholesterol & Lipid Disorders, Children	USPSTF	1996	Children and adolescents	Insufficient evidence to recommend for or against screening		
	GAPS	1994	Age > 2 years	See AAP/NCEP recommendations; measure cholesterol only once if normal.		
	AAP/NCEP	1992	Age > 2 years	Selective screening[a] every 5 years if normal[b] Fasting lipids if strong family history Random total cholesterol if a parent has total cholesterol > 240 mg/dL Clinician discretion (random total cholesterol) if unknown family history or presence of risk factors	Recommend pharmacologic treatment (eg, cholestyramine or cholestipol) if: (1) age > 10 years, on dietary therapy, and LDL > 190 mg/dL without other risk factors; or (2) LDL > 160 mg/dL and strong family history or 2 or more risk factors are present.[a]	Pediatrics 1992;89:525 Pediatrics 1992;90:469

CHOLESTEROL & LIPID DISORDERS, ADULTS

Disease Screening	Organization	Date	Population	Recommendations[a]	Comments	Source
Cholesterol & Lipid Disorders, Adults	NCEP III	2001	Men and women age > 20 years	Check fasting lipoprotein panel (if testing opportunity is non-fasting, use TC and HDL) every 5 years if in desirable range; otherwise see management algorithm[b]	NCEP III modifies recommendations (vs. NCEP II) to promote more aggressive primary prevention (ie, intensive lipid lowering) in persons with multiple risk factors for CHD.	JAMA 2001; 285:2486
	USPSTF	1996	Men ages 35–65 years Women ages 45–65 years	Random total cholesterol, periodicity based on risk factors; appropriate interval not known	Base treatment decisions on at least 2 cholesterol levels.	
			Men and women ages 66–75 years	Selective screening of older individuals with major CHD risk factors (hypertension, smoking, diabetes)		
			Men and women age > 75 years	Cholesterol screening not recommended		

CHOLESTEROL & LIPID DISORDERS, ADULTS

Disease Screening	Organization	Date	Population	Recommendations[a]	Comments	Source
Cholesterol & Lipid Disorders, Adults (continued)	ACP	1996	Men age < 35 years Women age < 45 years	Screening not recommended unless history or physical exam suggests familial lipoprotein disorder, or at least 2 other CHD risk factors are present	Recommendations were published before 2 large primary prevention trials with HMG-CoA reductase inhibitors demonstrated efficacy and safety. (Lancet 1994;344:1383, N Engl J Med 1995;333:1301) Base treatment decisions on at least 2 cholesterol levels.	Ann Intern Med 1996; 124:515
			Men ages 35–65 years Women ages 45–65 years	"Appropriate but not mandatory"; random total cholesterol every 5 years if normal		
			Men and women ages 66–75 years	Insufficient evidence to recommend for or against screening		
			Men and women age > 75 years	Screening not recommended		

CHOLESTEROL & LIPID DISORDERS, ADULTS

[a]AAP and NCEP recommend annual screening if strong family history (parents or grandparents) of cardiovascular events at or before age 55 years (MI, positive coronary angiogram, stroke, or peripheral vascular disease) or presence of "several" risk factors (cigarette smoking, hypertension, obesity, diabetes, lack of physical activity).

[b]Classify TC < 200 mg/dL as desirable, 200–239 mg/dL as borderline, or ≥ 240 mg/dL as high. Classify HDL < 40 as low, and ≥ 60 as high. Classify LDL < 100 as optimal, 100–129 as near or above optimal, 130–159 as borderline high, 160–189 as high, and ≥ 190 as very high.

If TC < 200 mg/dL and HDL ≥ 40 mg/dL, then repeat in 5 years; if TC ≥ 200 mg/dL or HDL < 40 mg/dL, then check fasting lipids and risk stratify based on LDL (see management algorithm).

DEMENTIA

Disease Screening	Organization	Date	Population	Recommendations	Comments	Source
Dementia	AHCPR	1996	Elderly	Perform selective screening[a] using a standardized instrument to assess cognitive function (see Mini Mental Status Exam in Appendix I).[b]	Screening instruments are useful for detecting multiple cognitive deficits and determining a baseline for future assessments. Reversible causes of dementia include vitamin B_{12} deficiency, neurosyphilis, and hypothyroidism. The additional benefit of identifying early dementia is to prepare family for future patient needs.	Ann Intern Med 1988;19:70 J Am Geriatr Soc 1988; 37:562 Activities of daily living: J Am Geriatr Soc 1985; 33:698 Mini-Mental Status Exam: J Psychiatr Res 1975;12:189
	USPSTF CTF	1996 1994	Elderly	Insufficient evidence to recommend for or against screening asymptomatic persons	Remain alert for signs of declining cognitive function.[a] Be aware of other causes of mental status changes, such as depression, delirium, medication effects, and coexisting illnesses.	

[a]Triggers that should initiate an assessment for dementia include difficulties in (1) learning and retaining new information, (2) handling complex tasks (eg, balancing a checkbook or cooking a meal), (3) reasoning ability (eg, a new disregard for social norms), (4) spatial ability and orientation (eg, difficulty driving or getting lost), (5) language (eg, difficulties in word-finding), and (6) behavior (eg, appearing more passive or more irritable than usual).

[b]DSM IV diagnosis of dementia requires: (1) evidence of decline in functional abilities and (2) evidence of multiple cognitive deficiencies.

DEPRESSION

Disease Screening	Organization	Date	Population	Recommendations	Comments	Source
Depression	GAPS Bright Futures	1994 1994	Adolescents	Annual screening for behaviors or emotions that might indicate depression or risk of suicide	Clues to depression include poor school performance, alcohol or drug use, and deteriorating parental or peer relationships. Clues to suicide risk include family dysfunction, physical and sexual abuse, substance abuse, history of recurrent or severe depression, and prior suicide attempt or plans.[a]	
	USPSTF	1996	Adults	Insufficient evidence to recommend for or against screening		
	AHCPR	1993	Adults	Selective screening when risk factors are present[b,c]	See screening instruments (Geriatric Depression Scale, Beck Depression Inventory Short Form, PRIME-MD) in Appendix I.	Clinical Practice Guideline No. 5: Depression in Primary Care. Agency for Healthcare Policy and Research; 1993. AHCPR Publication 93-0550 Arch Gen Psychiatry 1998;55:1121

DEPRESSION

[a]Suicide risk increases as the number of conditions increases. Parents of adolescents at risk for suicide should reduce access to firearms, weapons, or potentially lethal drugs in the home.

[b]Risk factors include prior episodes of depression, family history (first-degree relative) of depressive disorder, prior suicide attempts, age < 40 years, female gender, postpartum period, medical comorbidity, lack of social support, stressful life events, and current alcohol or substance abuse.

[c]Suspicion or documentation of depression by history should lead to a mental status exam that includes documentation of suicidal ideation; level of orientation, alertness, cooperation, and communication; level of motor activity; and presence or absence of psychotic features.

DIABETES MELLITUS

Disease Screening	Organization	Date	Population	Recommendations	Comments	Source
Diabetes Mellitus, Gestational	ADA	1998	Pregnant women age > 25 years or high risk[a]	Screening test: 1-hour OGTT at 24–28 weeks of gestation	Positive 1-hour OGTT: serum glucose > 140 mg/dL after 50 g oral glucose Confirmation test: 3-hour OGTT	Diabetes Care 1998;21 (suppl 1):1
	ACOG and AAP	1997	Pregnant women	Universal or selective screening at 24–28 weeks of gestation[b]		See Appendix IX
	USPSTF CTF	1996 1994	Pregnant women	Insufficient evidence to support screening	No evidence that universal screening results in meaningful clinical outcomes	

DIABETES MELLITUS

Disease Screening	Organization	Date	Population	Recommendations	Comments	Source
Diabetes Mellitus, Type 2	ADA	1998	Adults	Selective screening of high-risk adults with fasting glucose[c]	Positive test: fasting serum glucose > 126 mg/dL on 2 separate occasions Screening appears to be more cost-effective for younger people (ages 25–45 years) and blacks.	Diabetes Care 1998;21 (suppl 1):1 JAMA 1998;280:1757
	USPSTF CTF	1996 1994	Adults	Insufficient evidence to support screening asymptomatic adults		

[a]High risk is defined as either (1) obesity (BMI > 27 kg/m^2) + age < 25 years (see BMI Conversion Table in Appendix IV), (2) family history of diabetes in a first-degree relative, or (3) membership in one of the following ethnic groups: black, Hispanic, Native American, Asian American, or Pacific Islander.

[b]High risk is defined as maternal age > 30 years, family history of diabetes, previous macrosomia, malformed or stillborn infants, hypertension, glucosuria, or previous gestational diabetes.

[c]High risk is defined as either (1) age > 45 years; (2) family history of diabetes in parents or siblings; (3) membership in one of the following ethnic groups: black, Hispanic, Native American, Asian American, or Pacific Islander; (4) history of impaired fasting glucose, impaired glucose tolerance, gestational diabetes, or mother with infant birthweight > 9 lb; or (5) comorbid conditions, including hypertension (> 140/90 mm Hg) or dyslipidemia (HDL < 35 mg/dL or TGs > 250 mg/dL).

DOMESTIC VIOLENCE & ABUSE

Disease Screening	Organization	Date	Population	Recommendations	Comments	Source
Domestic Violence & Abuse	ACOG	1996	Women	Recommend routine, direct questions about domestic violence.	Controversy exists regarding the overall benefit of mandatory reporting of domestic violence. (JAMA 1995;273:1781) Barriers to screening include lack of provider education and time. Interventions that incorporated strategies in addition to provider education (eg, providing specific screening questions) were associated with significant increases in identification rates. (Am J Prev Med 2000;19:230)	
	ACOG	1996	Elderly		Some states have mandatory reporting of elder abuse and neglect.	

HEARING IMPAIRMENT

Disease Screening	Organization	Date	Population	Recommendations	Comments	Source
Hearing Impairment	AAP Joint Committee on Infant Hearing Bright Futures NIH	1999 1995 1994 1993	Normal-risk infants and children	All infants should be screened before 3 months of age with auditory brainstem response or otoacoustic emissions. Perform pure-tone audiometry at 3, 4, 5, 10, 12, 15, and 18 years of age.		Pediatrics 1995;95(1):152 Pediatrics 1999;103(2):527 NIH Consensus Statement 1993;11:1
	USPSTF CTF	1996 1994	Normal-risk infants and children	Insufficient evidence to recommend for or against routine screening of neonates. Routine screening beyond age 3 years is not recommended.		
	ASHA	1991	Normal-risk infants and children	Annual pure-tone audiometry for children functioning at a developmental level of age 3 years to grade 3		ASHA Suppl 1991;33:37
	USPSTF Joint Committee on Infant Hearing	1996 1995	High-risk infants and children[a,b]	Infants should be screened no later than 3 months of age. Screen infants and children < 2 years of age with increased risk. Screen every 6 months until 3 years of age if there is risk for delayed-onset hearing loss.		Pediatrics 1995;95(1):152

HEARING IMPAIRMENT

Disease Screening	Organization	Date	Population	Recommendations	Comments	Source
Hearing Impairment (continued)	AAP ASHA	1995 1990	High-risk children[b]	Children with frequent recurrent otitis media or middle-ear effusion, or both, should have audiology screening and monitoring of communication-skills development.		Pediatrics 1995;95(1):152 ASHA Suppl 1990;32:17
	AAFP AGS USPSTF ACOG CTF	2000 1997 1997 1996 1994	Adults	Question older adults periodically about hearing impairment, counsel about availability of hearing-aid devices, and make referrals for abnormalities when appropriate.		J Am Geriatr Soc 1997;45:344 http://www.aafp.org/exam/pos_gen_guide

[a]Increased neonatal risk: family history of hereditary sensorineural hearing loss, intrauterine infection, craniofacial anomalies, birthweight < 1500 g, hyperbilirubinemia requiring exchange transfusions, ototoxic medications, bacterial meningitis, Apgar scores 0–4 and 0–6, mechanical ventilation lasting > 5 days, and stigmata associated with a syndrome known to include hearing loss.

[b]Increased childhood risk: patient/caregiver concern regarding hearing, speech, language, or developmental delay; bacterial meningitis; head trauma associated with loss of consciousness or skull fracture; stigmata associated with a syndrome known to include hearing loss; ototoxic medications; recurrent or persistent otitis media with effusion; disorders affecting eustachian tube function; neurofibromatosis type 2; and neurodegenerative disorders. Delayed-onset hearing loss: as above for increased childhood risk plus family history of hereditary childhood hearing loss and intrauterine infection.

HEPATITIS B VIRUS

Disease Screening	Organization	Date	Population	Recommendations	Comments	Source
Hepatitis B Virus Infection, Chronic	USPSTF ACP ACIP	1996 1994 1993	Pregnant women	Screen all women with HBsAg[a] at first prenatal visit. Repeat in third trimester if woman is initially HBsAg negative and engages in high-risk behavior.[b]	Screening all pregnant women in the US each year is estimated to detect 22,000 HBsAg-positive mothers, and treatment of their newborns would prevent chronic HBV infection in 6000 neonates per year. (Pediatr Infect Dis J 1992;11:866)	MMWR 1991;40(RR-13):1 Int J Gynaecol Obstet 1993;40:172
	USPSTF ACP ACIP	1996 1994 1993	General population	Routine screening is not recommended.		
	USPSTF ACP ACIP	1996 1997 1994 1993	High-risk persons[b]	Insufficient evidence to recommend for or against screening to determine eligibility for vaccination, but recommendations for screening may be made based on cost-effectiveness analyses		

[a]Immunoassays for HBsAg have sensitivity and specificity > 98%. (MMWR 1993;42:707)

[b]High risk includes injection drug users, sexual contact with HBV-infected persons or with persons at high risk for HBV infection, multiple sexual partners, and male homosexual activity.

HEPATITIS C VIRUS

Disease Screening	Organization	Date	Population	Recommendations	Comments	Source
Hepatitis C Virus Infection, Chronic	CDC AAP	1998 1998	Persons at increased risk[a]	Perform routine counseling, testing, and appropriate follow-up.[b] See algorithm below.		MMWR 1998;47(RR-19):1 Pediatrics 1998;101(3):481

[a]Increased risk includes injection drug use, receipt of clotting factor concentrates before 1987, chronic hemodialysis, persistently abnormal ALT levels, receipt of blood from a donor who later tested positive for HCV, receipt of blood transfusion or blood components before July 1992, receipt of organ transplant before July 1992, health care workers after needle sticks or mucosal exposures to HCV-positive blood, and children born to HCV-positive women.

[b]Two types of tests are available for laboratory diagnosis of HCV infection: (1) detection of antibody to HCV antigens, and (2) detection and quantification of HCV nucleic acid. See algorithm below.

HCV INFECTION TESTING ALGORITHM FOR ASYMPTOMATIC PERSONS

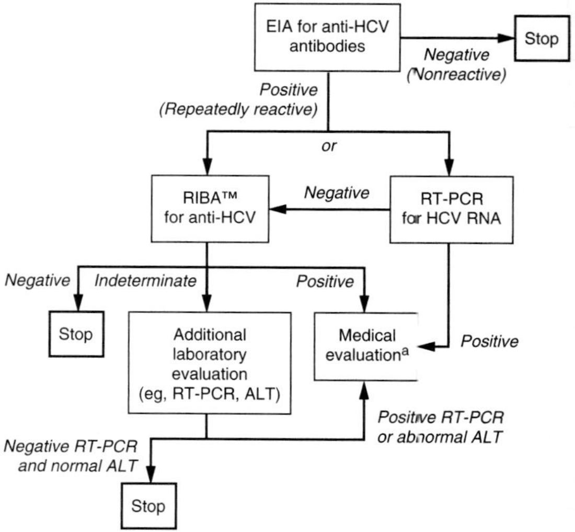

ALT = alanine aminotransferase; anti-HCV = antibody to HCV; EIA = enzyme immunoassay; RIBA™ = recombinant immunoblot assay; RT-PCR = reverse transcriptase polymerase chain reaction

[a]For possible anti-inflammatory and antiviral treatments.

Source: Adapted from MMWR 1998;47(RR-19):1.

HUMAN IMMUNODEFICIENCY VIRUS (HIV)

Disease Screening	Organization	Date	Population	Recommendations	Comments	Source
Human Immunodeficiency Virus	AAFP USPSTF Bright Futures GAPS CTF ACP AAP AMA CDC ACOG	2000 1996 1994 1994 1994 1994 1993 1993 1993 1992	People at increased risk[a]	Counseling and testing for HIV should be offered.	Initial screening test: EIA is considered reactive only when a positive result is confirmed in a second test of the original sample. Seroconversion is 95% within 6 months of infection. Specificity is > 99.5%. False-positives with EIA: nonspecific reactions in persons with immunologic disturbances (eg, systemic lupus erythematosus or rheumatoid arthritis), multiple transfusions, recent influenza, or rabies vaccination. Confirmatory testing is necessary using Western blot or indirect immunofluorescence assay. Home tests available.[b]	Pediatrics 1993;92:626 MMWR 1993;42 (RR-2):1 MMWR 1987;36:509 MMWR 1995;44 (RR-7):1 Ann Intern Med 1994;120:310 Pediatrics 1995;95(2):303 www.aafp.org/exam/pos_gen_guide.html AMA: HIV Blood Test Counseling. Physician Guidelines. 2nd ed. AMA, 1993.

HUMAN IMMUNODEFICIENCY VIRUS (HIV)

Disease Screening	Organization	Date	Population	Recommendations	Comments	Source
Human Immunodeficiency Virus (continued)	AAFP USPSTF ACOG AAP CDC	2000 1996 1996 1995 1995	Pregnant women	Counsel pregnant women about the potential benefit to their infant of early intervention for HIV and offer testing at first prenatal visit. Repeat testing in third trimester for women at high risk of recent exposure to HIV.[a]		Pediatrics 1995;95:303 N Engl J Med 1994;331:1173 http://www.aafp.org/exam/pos_gen_guide.html

[a]High risk: seeking treatment for STDs; male homosexual sex after 1975; past or present injection drug use; past or current exchange of sex for money or drugs; sex partners of people who are HIV-infected, bisexual, or injection drug users; or history of blood transfusion between 1978 and 1985.

[b]The FDA has approved 2 HIV home testing kits and warns about use of HIV home testing kits that have not been FDA approved. Consumers can obtain information about HIV home testing kits by calling the HIV/AIDS Program of the FDA in the Office of Special Health Issues at 301-827-4460. Health care provider follow-up is recommended for positive home HIV test results. (Oncology 1999;13(1):81)

HYPERTENSION, CHILDREN & ADOLESCENTS

Disease Screening	Organization	Date	Population	Recommendations	Comments	Source
Hypertension, Children & adolescents	USPSTF	1996	Age < 21 years	"During office visits"	Hypertension: BP > 95th percentile 3 different times within 1 month, adjusted for height (J Pediatr 1993;123:871) (see Appendix III) Major reason to screen children is early identification of conditions associated with hypertension (eg, coarctation of aorta, renal artery stenosis, renal parenchymal disease). Treatment: See[a] below.	Pediatrics 1987;79:1 Pediatrics 1996;98:649
	NHLBI	1996	Ages 3–20 years	Annual screening		
	Bright Futures	1994	Ages 3–21 years	Annual screening at ages 3–6, 8, and 10–21 years		
	GAPS	1994	Ages 11–18 years	Annual screening		

HYPERTENSION, ADULTS

Disease Screening	Organization	Date	Population	Recommendations	Comments	Source
Hypertension, Adults	JNC VI	1997	Age > 18 years	Annual screening If BP < 130/85 mm Hg, then every 2 years If BP 130–139/85–89 mm Hg, then annually If BP 140–159/90–99 mm Hg, then confirm within 2 months	Hypertension: SBP > 140 or DBP > 90 mm Hg Finger monitors are not accurate. (Fam Med 1996;61(50):53) Perform physical exam and routine labs.[b] Pursue secondary causes of hypertension.[c] Treatment: See[d,e] below.	Arch Intern Med 1997;157:2413
	AAFP USPSTF	2000 1996	Age > 21 years	Periodic screening If BP < 140/85 mm Hg, then every 2 years If DBP 85–89 mm Hg, then annually		http://www.aafp.org/exam/pos_gen_guide.html
	CTF	1994	Age > 21 years	BP screening at any visit		

HYPERTENSION, ELDERLY

Disease Screening	Organization	Date	Population	Recommendations	Comments	Source
Hypertension, Elderly	JNC VI	1997	Age > 60 years	Annual screening	Prevalence: 60–70% of persons > 60 years old Treatment[f] (JNC VI SBP goal < 140 mm Hg)	Hypertension 1995;25:305 N Engl J Med 1993;329:1912

[a]Treatment of primary (essential) hypertension in older children and adolescents is of unproved benefit; majority respond to weight loss and exercise. (Am J Cardiol 1983;52:763, Pediatrics 1978;61:245) The NHLBI recommends pharmacologic treatment of severe hypertension in addition to nonpharmacologic treatment (less than 1% of hypertensive children are classified as severe). (Arch Dis Child 1967;42:34)

[b]Physical exam should include: measurements of height, weight, and waist circumference; funduscopic exam (retinopathy); carotid auscultation (bruit); jugular venous pulsation; thyroid gland (enlargement); cardiac auscultation (left ventricular heave, S_3 or S_4, murmurs, clicks); chest auscultation (rales, evidence of chronic obstructive pulmonary disease); abdominal exam (bruits, masses, pulsations); exam of lower extremities (diminished arterial pulsations, bruits, edema); and neurologic exam (focal findings). Routine labs include urinalysis, complete blood count, electrolytes, creatinine, fasting glucose, lipids, and 12-lead electrocardiogram.

[c]Pursue secondary causes of hypertension when evaluation is suggestive (clues in parentheses) of: (1) pheochromocytoma (labile or paroxysmal hypertension accompanied by sweats, headaches, and palpitations), (2) renovascular disease (abdominal bruits), (3) autosomal dominant polycystic kidney disease (abdominal or flank masses), (4) Cushing's syndrome (truncal obesity with purple striae), (5) primary hyperaldosteronism (hypokalemia), (6) hyperparathyroidism (hypercalcemia), (7) renal parenchymal disease (elevated serum creatinine, abnormal urinalysis), (8) poor response to drug therapy, (9) well-controlled hypertension with an abrupt increase in blood pressure, (10) SBP > 180 or DBP > 110 mm Hg, or (11) sudden onset of hypertension.

[d]Treatment includes: (1) lifestyle modifications to affect blood pressure: Lose weight, limit alcohol to < 2 servings/d for men (< 1 serving/d for women), increase aerobic activity (30–45 min/d), reduce sodium intake (< 2.4 g of sodium or 6.0 g NaCl), maintain adequate dietary potassium (fruits and vegetables), and maintain adequate dietary calcium and magnesium. Note that the salt restriction recommendations are particularly applicable to black, elderly, and diabetic patients. (2) Lifestyle modifications to decrease heart disease risk: Reduce saturated fatty acid intake, trans-fatty acids, and dietary cholesterol; stop smoking.

HYPERTENSION, ELDERLY

[e]CHS/BHS pharmacologic treatment recommendations for DBP 90–99 mm Hg are dependent upon additional factors of target organ damage or diabetes. Otherwise, risk stratify according to higher pressures within the range, advanced age, male sex, smoking, dyslipidemia, or strong family history of cardiovascular disease. (BMJ 1993;306:983)

[f]Give pharmacy prescription if SBP > 160 mm Hg. Although SBP of 140–160 mm Hg is associated with greater cardiovascular morbidity, there is still no demonstration that pharmacologic therapy improves outcomes.

LEAD POISONING

Disease Screening	Organization	Date	Population	Recommendations	Comments	Source
Lead Poisoning	ACPM	2001	Infants and children	Selective screening at 12 months of high risk.[a]	Risk assessment should be performed during prenatal visits and continuing until 6 years of age.	Am J Prev Med 2001;20:78
	AAP CDC	1998 1997	Infants and children	Selective screening with blood lead level at 9–12 months, and again at 24 months when levels peak, of infants at high risk[b] Evaluation of blood lead level[c]	The Advisory Committee on Childhood Lead Poisoning Prevention (ACCLPP) includes Medicaid-enrolled children ages 1–5 years as high risk (MMWR 2000;49 (RR-14):1) CDC personal risk questionnaire: (1) Does your child live in or regularly visit a house (or other facility, eg, daycare) that was built before 1950? (2) Does your child live in or regularly visit a house built before 1978 with recent or ongoing renovations or remodeling (within the last 6 months)? (3) Does your child have a sibling or playmate who has or did have lead poisoning?	Pediatrics 1998; 101:1072 www.cdc.gov/nceh/programs/lead/guide/1997/guide97.htm
	AAFP USPSTF	1996	Infants at age 12 months	Selective screening with blood lead level for those infants at high risk[d]		

LEAD POISONING

[a]Criteria for being at high risk include: receipt of Medicaid or WIC, living in a community with ≥ 12% prevalence of elevated blood lead levels (BLLs) at ≥ 10 μg/mL; living in a community with ≥ 27% of homes built before 1950; or meeting 1 or more high risk criteria from a lead-screening questionnaire (see CDC comments above). Prevalence levels supported by recent cost-effectiveness studies (Arch Pediatr Adolesc Med 1998;152:1202).

[b]High risk of lead poisoning if any one of the following conditions exists: (1) Child lives in or regularly visits a house or child care facility built before 1950; (2) child lives in or regularly visits a house or child care facility built before 1978 that is being or has recently been renovated or remodeled (within the last 6 months); or (3) child has a sibling or playmate who has or did have lead poisoning.

[c]Confirm elevated lead levels with venous sample after screening sample from fingerstick: immediately if > 70 μg/mL, within 48 hours if 45–69 μg/mL, within 1 week if 20–44 μg/mL, and within 1 month if 10–19 μg/mL. See AAP guidelines for further treatment recommendations.

[d]Increased risk of lead poisoning exists for infants who: (1) live in communities in which the prevalence of lead levels requiring intervention is high or undefined, (2) live in or frequently visit a home built before 1950 with dilapidated paint or with recent or ongoing renovation or remodeling, (3) have close contact with a person who has an elevated lead level, (4) live near lead industry or heavy traffic, or (5) live with someone whose job or hobby involves lead exposure or who uses lead-based pottery or takes traditional remedies that contain lead.

OBESITY

Disease Screening	Organization	Date	Population	Recommendations	Comments	Source
Obesity	NHLBI NIDDKD	1998	Age > 18 years	Calculate BMI for all patients.[a]	The NHLBI makes a strong case for promoting weight loss in overweight individuals, particularly those with hypertension, diabetes, cardiovascular disease, and hyperlipidemia.	NHLBI Obesity Guidelines in Adults, 1998.
	AAFP USPSTF AAP Bright Futures GAPS	2000 1996 1994 1994	All age groups	Periodic height and weight measurements	Waist-hip ratio may also provide additional prognostic information beyond BMI and waist circumference. Among women 50–69 years of age free of cancer, heart disease and diabetes, waist-hip ratio best anthropometric predictor of total mortality. (Arch Intern Med 2000;160:2117)	www.aafp.org/exam/pos_gen_guide.html

[a]BMI is calculated as: weight (kg)/height (m) squared. See Appendix IV for BMI Conversion Table. Overweight is defined as BMI 25–29.9 kg/m^2 and obesity as BMI > 30 kg/m^2.

OSTEOPOROSIS

Disease Screening	Organization	Date	Population	Recommendations	Comments	Source
Osteoporosis	NIH	2001	Women	History and physical exam should evaluate for fracture risk. The value of universal screening with bone mineral densitometry (BMD) has not been established.	Until there is good evidence to support the cost-effectiveness of routine screening, or the efficacy of early initiation of preventive drugs, an individualized approach is recommended. A measurement of BMD should be considered when it will help the patient decide whether to institute treatment to prevent osteoporotic fracture.	JAMA 2001;285: 785–795
	NOF AAFP USPSTF ACOG AACE CTF ACP	1998 1997 1996 1996 1996 1994 1990	Women	Bone densitometry should not be routine. It should be considered for those at high risk of osteoporosis.[a]		Ann Intern Med 1990;112:516 Endocrine Practice 1996;2:155 http://www.nof.org http://www.aafp.org/exam/pos_gen_guide.html

[a]High risk: chronic steroid use (2 months or more), repeated fractures, early menopause, blood relative with osteoporosis, or known low bone mass or bone density. Bone densitometry may be useful to guide treatment in selected postmenopausal women.

OSTEOPOROSIS: SCREENING

SELECTIVE SCREENING FOR OSTEOPOROSIS IN PERSONS NOT CURRENTLY TAKING ANTI-OSTEOPOROSIS MEDICATIONS OR HAVING A HISTORY OF HIP FRACTURE
(Modified from the National Osteoporosis Foundation: Physician s guide to prevention & treatment of osteoporosis; Up To Date Screening for Osteoporosis by H.N. Rosen).

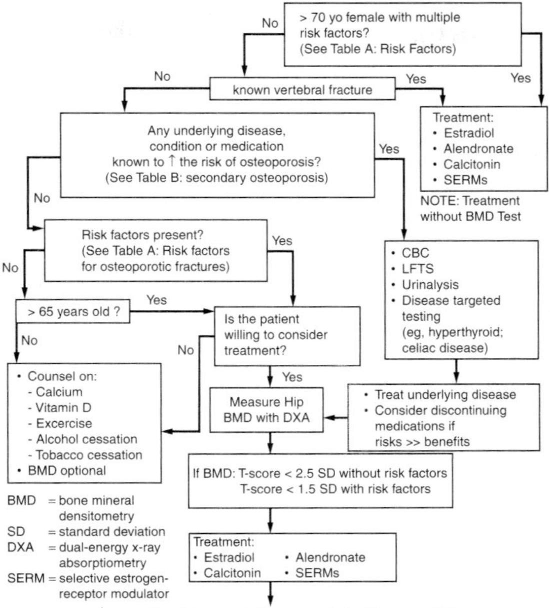

See Osteoporosis Management Algorithm, page 140

TABLE A: RISK FACTORS FOR OSTEOPOROTIC FRACTURE	
Potentially Modifiable	**Nonmodifiable**
Current cigarette smoker	**Personal history of fracture as an adult**
Low body weight (<127 lbs)	**History of fracture in first-degree relative**
Estrogen deficiency: -early menopause (age <45) of bilateral ovariectomy -prolonged premenopausal amenorrhea (>1 year)	Caucasian race
Low calcium intake (lifelong)	Advanced age
Alcoholism	Female sex
Impaired eyesight despite adequate correction	Dementia
Recurrent falls	Poor health/frailty
Inadequate physical activity	
Poor health/frailty	

Boldface items-personal or family history of Fracture, smoking, and low body weight-were Demonstrated in a large, ongoing, prospective US study to be key factors in determining the Risk of hip fracture (independent of bone Density).

National Osteoporosis Foundation.

Physician's guide to prevention and treatment of osteoporosis. Available at: http://www.nof.org/physguide/inside_cover.htm. Accessed January 18, 2001.

TABLE B: CAUSES OF GENERALIZED SECONDARY OSTEOPOROSIS IN ADULTS

Drugs	Endocrine Diseases or Metabolic Causes	Collagen Diseases	Nutritional Conditions	Other Causes
Aluminum	Acromegaly	Epidermolysis bullosa	Gastrectomy	Amyloidosis
Anticonvulsants	Adrenal atrophy and Addison's disease	Osteogenesis imperfecia	Malabsorption syndromes	Ankylosing spondylitis
Cigarette smoking	Congenital porphyria		Nutritional disorders	Chronic obstructive pulmonary disease
Cytotoxic drugs	Cushing's syndrome		Parenteral nutrition	Hemophilia
Excessive alcohol	Endometriosis		Pernicious anemia	Idiopathic scoliosis
Excessive thyroxine	Gonadal insufficiency (primary & secondary)		Severe liver disease (especially primary biliary cirrhosis)	Lymphoma & Leukemia
Glucocorticosteroids & adrenocorticotropin	Hemochromatosis			Mastocytosis
Gonadotropin-releasing hormone agonists	Hyperparathyroidism			Multiple myeloma
Heparin	Hyperphosphatemia			Multiple selerosis
Lithium	Diabetes mellitus type 1			Rheumatoid arthritis
Tamoxifen (premenopausal use)	Thyrotoxicosis			Sarcoidosis
	Tumor secretion of parathyroid hormone-related peptide			Thalassemia

National Osteoporosis Foundation.
Physician's guide to prevention and treatment of osteoporosis. Available at: http://www.nof.org/physguide/inside_cover.htm. Accessed January 18, 2001.

SCOLIOSIS

Disease Screening	Organization	Date	Population	Recommendations	Comments	Source
Scoliosis	USPSTF CTF	1996 1994	Adolescents	Insufficient evidence to recommend for or against routine screening of asymptomatic adolescents	Positive predictive value of bending test is 42.8% for scolioses of > 5 degrees and 6.4% for > 15 degrees; sensitivity 74%, specificity 78%. (Am J Public Health 1985;75:1377)	
	Bright Futures	1994	Adolescents	Screen during physical exam in adolescents and children > 8 years of age.		
	AAOS	1992	Adolescents	Screen girls twice (ages 10 and 12 years) and boys once (age 13 or 14 years).		www.aaos.org/ wordhtml/papers/ position/ scolios.htm
	Scoliosis Research Society	1986	Adolescents	Perform annual screening of all children ages 10–14 years.		Scoliosis Research Society: Scoliosis: A Handbook for Patients. Scoliosis Research Society, 1986.

SYPHILIS

Disease Screening	Organization	Date	Population	Recommendations	Comments	Source
Syphilis	AAFP AAP & ACOG USPSTF GAPS Bright Futures ACP	2000 1997 1996 1994 1994 1994 1986	Pregnant women and high-risk persons[a]	Screen all pregnant women with nontreponemal test (eg, RPR or VDRL) at first prenatal visit; repeat in third trimester and at delivery for women at high risk of acquiring infection during pregnancy. Screen high-risk (nonpregnant) persons with routine serologic test (nontreponemal test; eg, RPR or VDRL).	All reactive nontreponemal tests should be confirmed with a more specific treponemal test (eg, FTA-ABS). Perform follow-up serologic tests after treatment to document decline in titers (using the same test used initially). Sensitivity of nontreponemal tests varies with levels of antibodies: 62–76% in early primary syphilis, 100% during secondary syphilis, and 70% in untreated late syphilis. In late syphilis, previously reactive results revert to nonreactive in 25% of patients. Specificity of nontreponemal tests is 75–85% in persons with preexisting diseases or conditions (eg, collagen vascular diseases, injection drug use, advanced malignancy, pregnancy, malaria, tuberculosis, viral and rickettsial diseases) and 100% in persons without preexisting diseases or conditions.	Ann Intern Med 1986;104:368 Pediatrics 1994;94:568 MMWR 1993;42 (RR-14):1 http://www.aafp.org/exam/

[a]High risk includes commercial sex workers, persons who exchange sex for money or drugs, persons with other STDs (including HIV), and sexual contacts of persons with active syphilis.

THYROID DISEASE

Disease Screening	Organization	Date	Population	Recommendations	Comments	Source
Thyroid Disease	USPSTF	1996	Children and adults	Routine screening is not recommended.		
	ATA	2000	Women age ≥ 35 years	Screen with serum TSH at age 35 years, and every 5 years thereafter.	Individuals with symptoms and signs potentially attributable to thyroid dysfunction[aa] and those with risk factors for its development[bb] may require more frequent TSH testing. When there is suspicion of pituitary or hypothalamic disease, the serum FT4 concentration should be measured in addition to the serum TSH.	Arch Intern Med 2000;160:1573
	USPSTF	1996	Elderly	Insufficient evidence to recommend for or against screening	Clinicians should remain alert for subtle or nonspecific symptoms of hypothyroidism and maintain a low threshold for diagnostic evaluation using serum TSH. Controversy exists regarding Rx benefit for patients with subclinical hypothyroidism (elevated TSH; normal free thyroxine)	J Gen Intern Med 1996;11:744 Ann Intern Med 1984;101:18

THYROID DISEASE

Disease Screening	Organization	Date	Population	Recommendations	Comments	Source
Thyroid Disease (continued)	ACP	1991	Women age > 50 years	Perform selective screening for women with 1 or more general symptoms such as fatigue, weight gain, or depression.		Common Screening Tests. ACP, 1991.

[a]Increased risk of hypothyroidism among patients with autoimmune diseases, unexplained depression, cognitive dysfunction, or hypercholesterolemia.

[aa]Signs, symptoms and comorbidities suggestive of hypothyroidism include previous thyroid dysfunction; goiter; surgery or radiotherapy affecting the thyroid; diabetes mellitus; vitiligo; pernicious anemia; leukotrichia (prematurely gray hair); and medications (such as lithium carbonate and iodine-containing compounds, eg, amiodarone, radiocontrast agents, expectorants containing potassium iodide, and kelp).

[bb]Risk factors from family history include thyroid disease, pernicious anemia, diabetes mellitus and primary adrenal insufficiency. Laboratory test results suggestive of thyroid disease include hypercholesterolemia, hyponatremia, anemia, CPK and LDH elevations, hyperprolactinemia, hypercalcemia, alkaline phosphatase elevation, and hepatocellular enzyme elevation.

TUBERCULOSIS

Disease Screening	Organization	Date	Population	Recommendations	Comments	Source
Tuberculosis	AAFP USPSTF AAP CTF Bright Futures GAPS ATS	2000 1996 1996 1994 1994 1994 1992	Persons at increased risk of developing TB[a]	Screening by tuberculin skin test is recommended. Frequency of testing should be based on likelihood of further exposure to TB and level of confidence in the accuracy of the results.[b,c]	Persons with positive PPD test should receive chest x-ray and clinical evaluation for TB. If no evidence of active infection, provide INH prophylaxis if appropriate.	Am Rev Respir Dis 1992;146:1623 Pediatrics 1994;93:131 Pediatrics 1996;97:282 MMWR 1995;44(RR-11):19 www.aafp.org/exam.html

[a]Increased risk: persons infected with HIV, close contacts of persons with known or suspected TB (including health care workers), persons with medical risk factors associated with reactivation of TB (eg, silicosis, diabetes mellitus, prolonged corticosteroid therapy, end-stage renal disease, immunosuppressive therapy), immigrants from countries with high TB prevalence (eg, most countries in Africa, Asia, and Latin America), medically underserved and low-income populations, alcoholics, injection drug users, persons with abnormal chest x-rays compatible with past TB, and residents of long-term care facilities (eg, correctional institutions, mental institutions, nursing homes).

[b]Periodic (eg, ages 1, 4–6, and 6–11 years) tuberculin skin testing is recommended for children who live in high-prevalence regions or whose history for risk factors is incomplete or unreliable.

[c]Test: Give intradermal injection of 5 U of tuberculin PPD and examine 48–72 hours later. Criteria for positive skin test (diameter of induration): > 15 mm for low risk, > 10 mm for high risk (including children < 4 years of age), > 5 mm for very high risk (HIV, abnormal chest radiograph, recent contact with infected persons). If negative, consider 2-step testing to differentiate between booster effect and new conversion. Perform second test within 13 weeks. False-negative results occur in 5–10%, especially early in infection, with anergy, with concurrent severe illness, in newborns and infants < 3 months old, and with improper technique. Prior BCG vaccination is not considered a valid basis for dismissing positive results.

VISUAL IMPAIRMENT, GLAUCOMA & CATARACTS

Disease Screening	Organization	Date	Population	Recommendations	Comments	Source
Visual Impairment, Glaucoma & Cataracts	AAP Bright Futures AOA AAO	1996 1994 1994 1991	Infants and children	Eye and vision screening is recommended between birth and 2 months, at age 6 months, ages 3–5 years, and ages 5–6 years. AOA recommends continuing comprehensive eye and vision exams every 2 years thereafter.		Pediatrics 1996;98:153 www.aoanet.org/ia-need-exam.html www.eyenet.org
	AAFP USPSTF	2000 1996	Children	Vision screening for amblyopia and strabismus for all children once before entering school, preferably between ages 3 and 4 years Insufficient evidence to recommend for or against routine screening for decreased visual acuity among asymptomatic school children		www.aafp.org/exam/pos_gen_guide.html
	CTF	1994	Children	Eye and vision screening is recommended during periodic health exams.		

VISUAL IMPAIRMENT, GLAUCOMA & CATARACTS

Disease Screening	Organization	Date	Population	Recommendations	Comments	Source
Visual Impairment, Glaucoma & Cataracts (continued)	AAFP USPSTF CTF	1997 1996 1994	Adults	Insufficient evidence to recommend for or against routine eye and vision screening among asymptomatic nonelderly adults		www.aafp.org/exam.html
	AOA	1994	Adults	Comprehensive eye and vision exam every 2–3 years at ages 19–40 years, every 2 years at ages 41–60 years, and every 1 year at age > 61 years	Insufficient evidence to recommend for or against routine ophthalmoscopy or screening for elevated intraocular pressure or glaucoma by primary care physicians	www.aoanet.org/ia-regular-op-care.html
	AAO	1992	Adults	Comprehensive eye and vision exam every 35 years in blacks ages 20–39 years, and, regardless of race, every 2–4 years at ages 40–64 years and every 12 years beginning at age 65 years		www.eyenet.org
	AAFP AGS USPSTF CTF	2000 1997 1996 1994	Elderly	Perform routine eye and Snellen visual acuity screening. Optimal frequency is not known.		J Am Geriatr Soc 1997;45:344 http://www.aafp.org/exam/pos_gen_guide.html

2
Disease Prevention

BACILLE CALMETTE-GUÉRIN

Immunization	Organization	Date	Population	Recommendations	Comments	Source
Bacille Calmette-Guérin	USPSTF CDC ACIP ATS	1996 1996 1996 1992	Adults[a]	Vaccination with BCG is not recommended for adults in the United States.		Am Rev Respir Dis 1992;146:1623 MMWR 1996;45(RR-4): 1018

[a]Consider BCG for health care workers who work in settings in which: (1) A high percentage of TB patients are infected with *M. tuberculosis* resistant to both INH and rifampin; (2) transmission of such drug-resistant strains is likely; and (3) comprehensive infection control precautions have been implemented and have not been successful. Also use BCG for tuberculin-negative infants and children who cannot be placed on INH and who have continuous exposure to persons with active disease and those belonging to groups with a rate of new infections greater than 1% per year and for whom the usual surveillance and treatment programs may not be operationally feasible.

DIPHTHERIA-TETANUS-PERTUSSIS

Immunization	Organization	Date	Population	Recommendations	Comments	Source
Diphtheria-Tetanus-Pertussis	ACIP AAFP AAP ACPM	2001 2001 2001 1997	Infants and children	See Appendix V for recommended childhood immunization schedule	DTaP = diphtheria and tetanus toxoids and acellular pertussis vaccine, which has fewer side effects.	MMWR 2001; 50(1):7–10,19 www.aafp.org/exam/rep-520.html Am J Prev Med 1997;13(23):74
	USPSTF	1996	Infants and children	Administer DTP vaccine at ages 2, 4, and 6 months; DTP at 12–18 months or DTaP at 15–18 months; and DTP or DTaP between ages 4 and 6 years. Administer Td booster at ages 11–12 years (or 14–16 years).		

DIPHTHERIA-TETANUS-PERTUSSIS

Immunization	Organization	Date	Population	Recommendations	Comments	Source
Diphtheria-Tetanus-Pertussis (continued)	ACIP AAFP ACPM AGS ACOG ACP CTF	1999 2000 1998 1997 1996 1994 1994	Adults	Administer Td booster vaccination every 10 years or single booster at age 50 or 65 years.	If nonimmunized person is age > 7 years, administer 3 doses of Td. Give the second dose 48 weeks after the first, and administer the third dose 6–12 months after the second dose.	www.aafp.org/exam/table2.html ACOG: Guidelines for Women's Health Care. ACOG, 1996. ACP: Guide for Adult Immunization, 3rd ed. ACP, 1994. MMWR 1999;48:12 MMWR 1994; 43(RR-1): 1 J Am Geriatr Soc 1997;45:344 Am J Prev Med 1998; 14(2):156–158
	USPSTF	1996	Adults	All adults should receive a periodic Td booster (optimal interval not established, but standard regimen is every 10 years).		

HAEMOPHILUS INFLUENZAE TYPE B

Immunization	Organization	Date	Population	Recommendations	Comments	Source
***Haemophilus influenzae* Type B**	ACIP AAFP AAP ACPM USPSTF CTF	2001 2001 2001 1997 1996 1994	Infants and children	Conjugate vaccine at 2, 4, and 6 months, with a booster dose at 12–15 months. If PRP-OMP is used, a dose at 6 months is not required. CTF recommends booster dose given at 18 months.	Hib vaccination has high efficacy (>90%) for preventing Hib invasive disease. Since vaccine introduction, there has been a significant decline in the incidence of invasive *H. influenzae* disease. (Clinician's Handbook of Preventive Services, 2nd ed. International Medical Publishers, 1998)	MMWR 2001;50(1): 7–10,19 Am J Prev Med 1997; 13(23):74 http://www.aafp.org/exam/rep-520.html

HEPATITIS A VIRUS

Immunization	Organization	Date	Population	Recommendations	Comments	Source
Hepatitis A Virus	AAFP AAP ACIP USPSTF ACP	2001 2001 2001 1996 1994	Age > 2 years	Immunize high-risk individuals.[a,b]	If patient requires immediate protection against hepatitis A, administer immune globulin simultaneously with the first vaccine dose.	www.aafp.org/exam/rep-520.html Pediatrics 1996;98(6):1207 ACP: Guide for Adult Immunization, 3rd ed. ACP, 1994. MMWR 1999; 48(RR-12):1–37

[a]High risk: persons living in, traveling to, or working in areas where the disease is endemic and periodic outbreaks occur; institutionalized persons; men who have sex with men; injection drug users; military personnel; and certain hospital and laboratory workers. (See CDC traveler's web site at http://www.cdc.gov/travel.)

[b]Schedule: For age < 18 years, 3 doses, with second and third doses given 1 and 6–12 months after the first dose; for age > 18 years, 2 doses, with second dose at 6–12 months.

HEPATITIS B VIRUS

Immunization	Organization	Date	Population	Recommendations	Comments	Source
Hepatitis B Virus	ACIP AAFP AAP ACPM USPSTF	2001 2001 2001 1997 1996	Infants, children, and adolescents	Immunize all infants, and all children and adolescents not previously immunized.[a,b]		MMWR 2001;50(1):7–10,19 Am J Prev Med 1997;13(23):74 Pediatrics 1997;99(3):479 MMWR 1991;40(RR-13):1 http://www.aafp.org/exam/rep-520.html
	USPSTF AAFP	1996 2000	Young adults High-risk adults[c]	Immunize all young adults not previously vaccinated.[d] Immunize high-risk groups.[d]	Consider testing antibody response in individuals at very high risk of hepatitis B who are likely to have inadequate antibody response (ie, chronic renal dialysis patients, injection drug users, those with HIV infection).	http://www.aafp.org/exam/table2.html http://www.aafp.org/exam/table4.html

HEPATITIS B VIRUS

[a]Schedule: Immunize at ages 0–2 months, then 12 months after the first dose, then at ages 6–18 months. After infancy, give first dose, followed by second and third doses at 1 and 6 months.

[b]Infants of HBsAg-negative mothers should receive the 1st dose of Hep B vaccine by age 2 months. The 2nd dose should be at least 1 month after the first. The 3rd dose should be at least 4 months after the first dose and at least 2 months after the second dose, but not before age 6 months. Infants of HBsAg-positive mothers: Give hepatitis B vaccine and hepatitis B immune globulin (0.5 mL) within 12 hours of birth. The 2nd dose is recommended at 1–2 months of age, and the 3rd dose at age 6 months. Infants for whom maternal HBsAg status is unknown: Give hepatitis B vaccine within 12 hours of birth and determine maternal HBsAg status: If HbsAg is positive, the infant should receive hepatitis B immune globulin as soon as possible (no later than age 1 week).

[c]High risk: men who have had sex with men, injection drug users and their sexual partners, history of sexual activity with multiple partners or history of another STD, international travelers to countries where HBV is of high or intermediate endemicity, recipients of certain blood products (including hemodialysis patients), and persons in health-related jobs with frequent exposure to blood or blood products.

[d]Recommended regimen: initial vaccine, then repeat at 1 and 6 months.

INFLUENZA

Immunization	Organization	Date	Population	Recommendations	Comments	Source
Influenza	AAFP ACIP AGS USPSTF ACP CTF	2000 2000 1997 1996 1994 1994	Ages 6 months to 64 years	Administer annually to high-risk persons.[a,b]	Influenza vaccination has also been shown to decrease work loss days in otherwise healthy, nonelderly adults. (N Engl J Med 1995;333:889)	http://www.aafp.org/exam/table2.html http://www.aafp.org/exam/table4.html MMWR 2000;49(RR-3):1–28. ACP: Guide for Adult Immunization, 3rd ed. ACP, 1994. http://www.cdc.gov/ncidod/diseases/flu/fluvirus.html
	ACOG	1996	Women age >60 years	Administer annually.		
	AAFP ACIP	2000	Age >50 years	Administer annually.		http://www.aafp.org/exam/table2.html MMWR 2000;49(RR-3):1–28. http://www.cdc.gov/ncidod/diseases/flu/fluvirus.html
	AGS USPSTF ACP CTF	1997 1996 1994 1994	Age >65 years	Administer annually.		J Am Geriatr Soc 1997;45:344 www.aafp.org/exam/app-d_c.html MMWR 1997;46(RR-9):1 ACP: Guide for Adult Immunization, 3rd ed. ACP, 1994.

INFLUENZA

Immunization	Organization	Date	Population	Recommendations	Comments	Source
Influenza (continued)	ACP	1994	Health care providers and household members of high-risk persons[a]	Administer annually.		ACP: Guide for Adult Immunization, 3rd ed. ACP, 1994.

[a]High risk: residents of chronic care facilities and persons with chronic cardiopulmonary disorders, metabolic diseases (including diabetes mellitus), hemoglobinopathies, immunosuppression, or renal dysfunction or health care providers for these patients.

[b]Although influenza vaccine is the primary way to prevent influenza, antiviral drugs are an important adjunct to vaccine for the control and prevention of influenza. Four currently approved antiviral medications are available in the United States: amantadine, rimantadine, zanamivir, and oseltamivir. Amantadine and rimantadine are approved for the chemoprophylaxis and treatment of influenza A infection only. Zanamivir and oseltamivir are neuraminidase inhibitors with activity against both influenza A and B viruses. When administered prophylactically to healthy adults or children, both amantadine and rimantadine are 60–90% effective in preventing illness from influenza A infection; oseltamivir is approximately 60–90% effective in preventing illness from influenza infection. Chemoprophylaxis is not a substitute for vaccination, but may be considered in the following situations: 1) protection of high-risk persons who have been vaccinated after influenza activity has begun. The time from vaccination until development of protective antibody levels is approximately 2 weeks; 2) protection of high-risk persons who cannot receive influenza vaccine because of allergies or other contraindications; 3) protection of unvaccinated close contacts of persons at high risk for complications from influenza during the peak of the influenza season to reduce the spread of influenza to high-risk persons; 4) protection of immunocompromised persons who may not develop protective levels of antibody following vaccination; 5) control of outbreaks in an institution housing or caring for high-risk people. (http://www.cdc.gov/ncidod/disease/flu/fluvirus.html)

MEASLES-MUMPS-RUBELLA

Immunization	Organization	Date	Population	Recommendations	Comments	Source
Measles-Mumps-Rubella	ACIP AAFP AAP ACPM USPSTF	2001 2001 2001 1997 1996	Children	Administer at ages 12–15 months and again at 4–6 years of age; 11–12 years is an acceptable alternative for second dose.	Children age >6 years who have not yet received 2 doses should be vaccinated, with the goal that all children will have had 2 doses of MMR vaccine by ages 11–12.	MMWR 2001;50(1):7–10,19 Am J Prev Med 1997;13:74 Clinician's Handbook of Preventive Services, 2nd ed. International Medical Publishing, 1998. Pediatrics 1998;101(1):129 www.aafp.org/exam/rep-520.html Am J Prev Med 1997;13(23):74
	AAFP ACPM	2000 1998	Adults born after 1956 who lack evidence of immunity	Two doses recommended for individuals in college settings and health care workers (2nd dose at least 1 month after 1st).	Evidence of immunity: receipt of live vaccine on or after 1st birthday, laboratory evidence of immunity, hx of physician-diagnosed measles.	http://www.aafp.org/exam/pos_spec_sta.html http://www.aafp.org/exam.table4.html Am J Prev Med 1998;14(2):156–158

MEASLES-MUMPS-RUBELLA

Immunization	Organization	Date	Population	Recommendations	Comments	Source
Measles-Mumps Rubella (continued)	AAFP USPSTF ACOG ACP CTF ACIP	2000 1996 1996 1994 1994 1994	Women of childbearing age	Obtain history of vaccination and serology, or offer vaccination (for rubella).	Do not administer rubella vaccine to pregnant women. Women receiving vaccine should not become pregnant for 3 months after vaccination.	http://www.aafp.org/exam/table4.html ACP: Guide for Adult Immunization, 3rd ed. ACP, 1994. MMWR 1994;43(RR-1):1
	ACP	1994	Health care workers	ACP recommends documentation of serologic immunity or vaccination of all health care workers.		ACP: Guide for Adult Immunization, 3rd ed. ACP, 1994.

POLIOMYELITIS VIRUS

Immunization	Organization	Date	Population	Recommendations	Comments	Source
Poliomyelitis Virus	ACIP AAFP AAP	2001 2001 2001	Infants and children	An all-inactivated poliovirus vaccine (IPV) schedule is recommended for routine childhood polio vaccination in the United States. All children should receive 4 doses of IPV at 2 months, 4 months, 6–18 months, and 4–6 years of age. Oral poliovirus vaccine (OPV) should be used only in selected circumstances.		MMWR 2000; 49(RR-5):1–22 http://www.aafp.org/exam/rep-520.html MMWR 2001; 50(1):7–10,19
	ACPM USPSTF	1997 1996	Infants and children	Give OPV at ages 2 months, 4 months, 6–18 months, and 4–6 years.		Am J Prev Med 1997;13(23):74

STREPTOCOCCUS PNEUMONIAE

Immunization	Organization	Date	Population	Recommendations	Comments	Source
Streptococcus pneumoniae	AAFP AAP ACIP	2001 2001 2001	Children	The heptavalent conjugate pneumococcal vaccine (PCV)(Prevnar) is recommended for all children 2–23 months of age. It is also recommended for certain children 24–59 months of age. PCV is normally administered as a series of 4 inoculations given at 2, 4, 6 and 12–15 months of age (see Appendix V).	PCV is not indicated for use in adult patients or as a substitute for other approved pneumococcal polysaccharide vaccines that are approved for use in high-risk children more than 2 years of age.	MMWR 2000; 49(RR-9):1–35. MMWR 2001;50(1):7–10,19 http://www.aafp.org/policy/camp/24.html
	ACPM AAFP ACIP USPSTF ACOG ACP	1998 1997 1997 1996 1996 1994	Ages 2–64 years	Immunize high-risk persons.[a]	Routine revaccination is not recommended but may be appropriate and is safe in individuals at highest risk for morbidity and mortality from pneumococcal disease who were vaccinated > 5 years previously or if age was < 65 years at the time of primary vaccination. (MMWR 1997;46(RR-8):1)	www.aafp.org/exam/table4.html ACP: Guide for Adult Immunization, 3rd ed. ACP, 1994. MMWR 1997; 46(RR-8):1 Am J Prev Med 1998;14(2):156–158

STREPTOCOCCUS PNEUMONIAE

Immunization	Organization	Date	Population	Recommendations	Comments	Source
***Streptococcus pneumoniae* (continued)**	CTF	1994	Age > 55 years	Insufficient evidence to recommend for or against immunization for immunocompetent individuals age > 55 years living independently. Good evidence to recommend for immunocompetent individuals age > 55 years living in institutions and patients with history of sickle cell disease or history of splenectomy.	Immunization	
	AAFP AGS ACIP USPSTF ACOG ACP	2000 1997 1997 1996 1996 1994	Age ≥ 65 years	Recommended for all individuals age ≥ 65 years.		J Am Geriatr Soc 1997;45:344 www.aafp.org/exam/table2.html MMWR 1997;46(RR-8):1 ACP: Guide for Adult Immunization, 3rd ed. ACP, 1994.

[a]Increased risk: institutionalized persons age > 50 years, chronic cardiac or pulmonary disease, diabetes mellitus, anatomic asplenia, special environments with increased risk of pneumococcal disease (eg, certain Native American and Alaska Native populations), alcoholism, cirrhosis, chronic renal failure, nephrotic syndrome, sickle cell disease, multiple myeloma, metastatic or hematologic malignancy, and acquired or congenital immunodeficiency.

VARICELLA VIRUS

Immunization	Organization	Date	Population	Recommendations	Comments	Source
Varicella Virus	ACIP AAFP AAP ACPM USPSTF	2001 2001 2001 1997 1996	Children[a]	Give 1 dose at any visit on or after the first birthday for susceptible children (lacking reliable history or never immunized).	Consider offering serologic testing to adolescents and adults without reliable history of infection or immunization.	MMWR 2001;50(1):7–10,19 Am J Prev Med 1997;13(23):74 Pediatrics 1995;95(5):791 MMWR 1996;45(RR-11):1
	ACIP AAFP AAP ACPM USPSTF	2001 2001 2001 1997 1996	Persons age >13 years with unknown history of childhood chickenpox	Give 2 doses at least 4 weeks apart.[b]		MMWR 2001;50(1):7–10,19 Am J Prev Med 1997;13(23):74 Pediatrics 1995;95(5):791 MMWR 1996;45(RR-11):1 http://www.aafp.org/exam/table2.html

[a]Varicella vaccine should not be given routinely to immunocompromised individuals. The presence of an immunodeficient household contact does not contraindicate vaccine use in other household members.

[b]Loss of immunity to varicella may wane after vaccination, but no evidence of loss of immunity has been noted in 6–10 years of follow-up while wild-type varicella continues to circulate. As a result of widespread but not universal use of vaccine, an increased rate of clinical cases of varicella could occur in adults who were not vaccinated as children.

BREAST CANCER

Disease	Organization	Date	Population	Recommendations	Comments	Source
Breast Cancer	NCI	2001	Women	Avoid unnecessary breast irradiation. Low-fat diet and exercise may decrease risk. Genetic Screening: Little evidence to support or quantify potential beneficial effect of genetic screening (*BRCA1*/*BRCA2*) Tamoxifen: Risks and benefits have to be weighed, and decisions regarding use of tamoxifen for prevention must be individualized.	Less than 50% of all breast cancer cases are attributable to well-established risk factors; many risk factors are not modifiable. A RCT has shown that tamoxifen reduces the risk of developing breast cancer in women at increased risk. Tamoxifen also increases the risk of endometrial cancer and of thrombotic vascular events (J Natl Cancer Inst 1998;90:1371).	http://cancernet.nci.nih.gov

BREAST CANCER

Disease	Organization	Date	Population	Recommendations	Comments	Source
Breast Cancer (continued)				HRT: Patients considering HRT should weigh its potential effect on breast cancer against evidence that it reduces overall mortality. Mastectomy: Because of the physical and psychological effects and the irreversibility of the procedure, decisions regarding this option must be considered on an individual basis.	The use of hormone replacement therapy (HRT) with estrogen alone or in combination with progesterone may be associated with increased risk of developing breast cancer. This risk may be proportionate to duration of use and related to combination therapy. Bilateral prophylactic mastectomy is associated with a reduction in risk of breast cancer by as much as 90% among women with an increased risk of breast cancer due to a strong family history.	

BREAST CANCER

Disease	Organization	Date	Population	Recommendations	Comments	Source
Breast Cancer (continued)	ASCO	1999	Women at high risk[a]	For women with a 5-year projected risk of breast cancer of >1.66%, tamoxifen (at 20 mg/d for up to 5 years) may be offered to reduce their risk. Tamoxifen use should be discussed as part of an informed decision-making process, with careful consideration of risks and benefits. Premature to recommend raloxifene use to lower the risk of developing breast cancer outside of a clinical trial setting.[b]	Women being considered for tamoxifen therapy should be evaluated by health care providers familiar with evaluation of individual breast cancer risk and the risks and benefits of tamoxifen use. Currently insufficient evidence to determine whether tamoxifen provides overall health benefit or increased breast cancer-specific or overall survival.	www.asco.org J Clin Oncol 1999;17(6):1939

[a]Predicted risk of breast cancer calculated by using the Gail model, which considers age, number of first-degree relatives with breast cancer, number of previous breast biopsies, age at first live birth, and age at menarche. (J Natl Cancer Inst 1999;91:1829)

[b]Among postmenopausal women with osteoporosis, the risk of invasive breast cancer was decreased by 75% during 3 years of treatment with raloxifene. (JAMA 1999; 281(23):2189) The Study of Tamoxifen and Raloxifene (STAR) began recruiting volunteers in May 1999. This study will compare tamoxifen and raloxifene for their effects on reduction of breast cancer development in postmenopausal women. Information is available from http://cancertrials.nci.nih.gov/ or from the National Cancer Institute's Cancer Information Service (1-800-422-6237).

ENDOCARDITIS

Disease	Organization	Date	Population	Recommendations	Comments	Source
Endocarditis	AHA	1997	High-risk persons[a] Moderate-risk persons[b]	Give antibiotic prophylaxis[c] before bacteremia-producing procedures.[d,e]		JAMA 1997;277:1794

[a]Patients at high risk for endocarditis include those with prosthetic heart valves (including bioprosthetic and homograft valves), previous bacterial endocarditis, complex cyanotic congenital heart disease (including single ventricle states, transposition of the great arteries, tetralogy of Fallot), and surgically constructed systemic pulmonary shunts or conduits.

[b]Patients at moderate risk for endocarditis include those with most other congenital heart diseases (excluding isolated secundum atrial septal defect and surgically repaired atrial septal defect, ventricular septal defect, or patent ductus arteriosus without residua beyond 6 months), acquired valvular dysfunction (eg, rheumatic heart disease), hypertrophic cardiomyopathy, and mitral valve prolapse with valvular regurgitation or thickened leaflets.

[c]Standard prophylaxis regimen for dental, oral, respiratory tract, or esophageal procedures: amoxicillin (adults 2.0 g; children 50 mg/kg orally 1 hour before procedure). If unable to take oral medications, give ampicillin (adults 2.0 g IM or IV; children 50 mg/kg IM or IV within 30 minutes of procedure). If penicillin-allergic, give clindamycin (adults 600 mg; children 20 mg/kg orally 1 hour before procedure) or cephalexin or cefadroxil (adults 2.0 g; children 50 mg/kg orally 1 hour before procedure) or azithromycin or clarithromycin (adults 500 mg; children 15 mg/kg orally 1 hour before procedure). If penicillin-allergic and unable to take oral medications, give clindamycin (adults 600 mg; children 20 mg/kg IV within 30 minutes before procedure) or cefazolin (adults 1 g; children 25 mg/kg IM or IV within 30 minutes of procedure). See reference for recommended antibiotic regimens for other procedures. (JAMA 1997;277:1794)

[d]Bacteremia-producing procedures include: (1) dental and oral procedures including dental extractions, periodontal procedures, dental implant placement and reimplantation of avulsed teeth, endodontic (root canal) instrumentation, subgingival placement of antibiotic fibers or strips, initial placement of orthodontic bands but not brackets, intraligamentary local anesthetic injections, and prophylactic cleaning of teeth or implants where bleeding is anticipated; (2) respiratory tract procedures including tonsillectomy and adenoidectomy, surgical operations involving the respiratory mucosa, and bronchoscopy with a rigid bronchoscope; and (3) genitourinary tract procedures including prostatic surgery, cystoscopy, and urethral dilation.

[e]Prophylaxis for high-risk but not moderate-risk patients is recommended for patients undergoing gastrointestinal tract procedures including sclerotherapy, esophageal stricture dilation, ERCP with biliary obstruction, biliary tract surgery, and surgical operations involving the intestinal mucosa.

MYOCARDIAL INFARCTION

Disease	Organization	Date	Population	Recommendations	Comments	Source
Myocardial Infarction	AHA	1997	All	Dietary guidelines: (1) consume a variety of fruits and vegetables; choose 5 or more servings per day. (2) consume a variety of grain products, including whole grains; choose 6 or more servings per day. Exercise regularly: 3–4 times per week for 30 minutes. Control weight: achieve and maintain BMI at 21–25 kg/m^2 (see Appendix IV). Strongly encourage smoking cessation.	Based on the Nurses' Health Study, women adhering to all 4 recommendations had a relative risk of coronary events of 0.17 compared to all other women (N Engl J Med 2000;343:16).	Circulation 1997;95:23 Circulation 2000;102: 2284
	AHA	1997	Hyperlipidemia	Primary prevention of MI includes diet[a] and HMG-CoA reductase inhibitors in patients without a history of CHD and < 2 CHD risk factors[c] (goal LDL < 160 mg/dL) or >2 CHD risk factors (goal LDL < 130 mg/dL).[b] For screening recommendations, see page 34; also see new NCEP III screening and management (page 124) recommendations.	Short-term reduction in LDL using dietary counseling by dietitians is superior to that achieved by physicians (Am J Med 2000;109:549). RCTs have demonstrated the CHD and mortality benefit and safety of treatment of patients with hypercholesterolemia (pravastatin 40 mg/d) (N Engl J Med 1995;333:1301) and the CHD benefit of treatment of average cholesterol and LDL levels (but low HDL) (lovastatin 20–40 mg/d). (JAMA 1998;279:1615)	Circulation 1997;95: 2330

MYOCARDIAL INFARCTION

Disease	Organization	Date	Population	Recommendations	Comments	Source
Myocardial Infarction (continued)	AHA	1997	Hypertension	BP goal: < 140/90 mm Hg. See page 128 for JNC VI treatment algorithms.	Since JNC VI (1997), RCTs now support all 4 major drug classes as first-line therapy for hypertension. Meta-analysis suggests that beta-blockers should not be first-line therapy for uncomplicated hypertension in persons age > 60 years. (JAMA 1998;279:1903)	Arch Intern Med 1997;157: 2413
	AHA	1997	Diabetes	Treat diabetes to achieve HbA1c < 1 unit above normal (see page 131 for diabetes treatment algorithm).	ACE inhibitors should be first choice for diabetics with hypertension. (N Engl J Med 1998;338:645, BMJ 1998;317:703, Diabetes Care 1998;21:597) Studies are supporting more aggressive BP control in this population (eg, < 130/80 mm Hg). (Lancet 1998;351:1755)	Arch Intern Med 1997;157: 2413

[a]AHA recommends (1) limit intake of foods with a high content of cholesterol-raising fatty acids [saturated (sources: full fat dairy products, fatty meats, tropical oils)] and trans-fatty acids (sources: commercially available fried foods; some margarines) to achieve a goal of < 10% calories from cholesterol-raising fatty acids, (2) limit the intake of foods high in cholesterol to achieve a goal of < 300 mg/day, and (3) substitute grains and unsaturated fatty acids from fish, vegetables, legumes, and nuts (Circulation 2000;102:2284).

[b]Reviews of current studies suggest that reducing cholesterol levels beyond target levels, in patients without diabetes, is not justified. (Ann Intern Med 2000;133:549).

[c]CHD risk factors include age (men > 44 years, women > 54 years or postmenopausal), hypertension, diabetes, smoking, HDL < 35 mg/dL, and family history of CHD in first-degree relatives (male relatives < 55 years, female relatives < 65 years). If HDL is > 60 mg/dL, subtract 1 risk factor from number of positive risk factors.

OSTEOPOROSIS

Disease	Organization	Date	Population	Recommendations	Comments	Source
Osteoporosis	NIH NOF AAFP USPSTF ACOG AACE CTF ACP	2001 2000 2000 1996 1996 1996 1994 1990	Women	Counsel all women about potential benefits and risks of hormone prophylaxis (HRT) and about fracture risk reduction (dietary calcium, vitamin D, weight-bearing exercise, smoking cessation, moderate alcohol intake).[a] Predictors of low bone mass include increased age, estrogen deficiency, white race, low weight and body mass index (BMI), family history of osteoporosis, smoking, history of prior fractures. Use of alcohol and caffeine-containing beverages is inconsistently associated with decreased bone mass. Grip strength and current exercise are associated with increased bone mass.	An estrogen-progestin regimen may increase breast cancer risk (increased RR = 0.12 per year of treatment) beyond that associated with estrogen alone (increased RR = 0.03 per year of treatment) among women with BMI $\leq$ 24.4 kg/m^2. (JAMA 2000;283:485) Medical disorders associated with osteoporosis include hypogonadism (men), use of glucocorticoids, thyroid hormone excess, anticonvulsant therapy, hypercalciuria, hyperparathyroidism, and malabsorption.	JAMA 2001;285:785–795 Endocrine Practice 1996;2:155 http://www.nof.org http://www.aafp.org/

[a]Recommended HRT: 0.625 mg conjugated estrogen or equivalent once daily; for women with a uterus, add 2.5 mg medroxy progesterone acetate (MPA) or equivalent daily or 510 mg MPA daily for 10–14 days each month to decrease the risk of endometrial cancer. Raloxifene, a selective estrogen-receptor modulator (SERM), has been shown to reduce the risks of vertebral fracture by 36% in large clinical trials. For women unable to tolerate estrogen who are at high risk for fracture, consider alendronate or risedronate. Recommended calcium: teens to 20s, 1200 mg/d; 20s to menopause, 1000 mg/d; postmenopause, 1500 mg/d. Recommended vitamin D: 400–600 IU/day. (NIH Consensus Statement 1994;12:1)

OSTEOPOROSIS: PREVENTION

ALL ♀ AT RISK INDIVIDUALS*

↓

COUNSEL ON:

1. Tobacco cessation
2. Limit alcohol intake
3. Regular weight bearing exercise ≥30 min. 3x/wk
   Muscle strengthening exercise
4. Adequate Ca^{2+} intake 1000–1500 mg/d
   Adequate vitamin D 800 IU/d
5. Consider estrogen replacement

PREMENOPAUSAL/ PERIMENOPAUSAL

- Identify estrogen-deficient with ↓ bone mass & institute treatment to preserve bone mass
- Adjust thyroid dose if needed to avoid over-replacement

POSTMENOPAUSAL

- Identify and treat those ♀ with very low bone mineral density, sensory deficits, neurologic disease & arthritis, all of which can lead to ↑ frequency of falls
- Adjust drug dosages for drugs that are sedating, slow reflexes, ↓ coordination & impair a person's ability to break impact of a fall
- Gait & balance training to ↓ risk of falls

ELDERLY

- See postmenopausal recommendations; in addition:
  - Anchor rugs
  - Minimize clutter
  - Remove loose wires
  - Use non-skid mats
  - Handrails in halls bathrooms & stairwells
  - Adequate lighting in halls, stairwells & entrances
  - Wear sturdy low heeled shoes

(Adapted from AACE clinical practice guidelines for the prevention & treatment of postmenopausal osteoporosis)

*See page 91 for description of risks.

STROKE

Disease	Organization	Date	Population	Recommendations	Comments	Source
Stroke	JNC VI	1997	Hypertension	See page 52 for screening and diagnosis recommendations. See page 131 for JNC VI hypertension management algorithm.	JNC VI approach endorsed by AHA (Circulation 2001;103:163)	Arch Intern Med 1997;157:2413
	AHA	2001	Atrial fibrillation	Age < 65 years, no risk factors: aspirin Age < 65 years, w/risk factors:[a] warfarin (INR 2.0–3.0) Age 65–75 years, no risk factors: aspirin or warfarin Age 65–75 years w/risk factors: warfarin (INR 2.0–3.0) Age > 75 years: warfarin (INR 2.0–3.0) See pages 113–114 for atrial fibrillation management algorithm.	Average stroke rate about 5% per year (in those with no Hx of stroke or TIA). Meta-analysis concluded that adjusted-dose warfarin reduced the absolute risk of stroke by about 2.7% per year (NNT = 37) compared with 1.5% reduction for aspirin (NNT = 67). Risk of major bleed = 0.6% per year (NNH = 167); risk of intracranial bleed = 0.3% per year (NNH = 333). (Ann Intern Med 1999; 131:492)	Circulation 2001;103:163.

STROKE

Disease	Organization	Date	Population	Recommendations	Comments	Source
Stroke (continued)	ACCP	1995	Atrial fibrillation	Give anticoagulation with warfarin; target prothrombin time INR = 2.0–3.0. All patients with > 1 risk factor for stroke:[b] Give warfarin as above. Age < 65 years and no risk factors: Give no treatment or aspirin. Age > 65 years and no risk factors: Give aspirin or oral anticoagulants.		Chest 1995;108:Suppl.
	ACP	1994	Atrial fibrillation	Similar to ACCP, except uses age 60 years as cutoff for no risk factors		Ann Intern Med 1994;121:54
	AHA	2001	Diabetes	Improve glucose control and treat hypertension. Refer to USPSTF and ADA for screening and treatment.		Circulation 2001;103:163.
	AHA CNS USPSTF CTF SVS	2001 1997 1996 1994 1992	Carotid arterx sterosis	See page 31 for screening and treatment guidelines. Clear consensus exists on efficacy of treatment for symptomatic CAS; treatment of asymptomatic CAS is controversial.		Circulation 2001;103:163. CMAJ 1997;157:653 J Vasc Surg 1992; 15:469

STROKE

Disease	Organization	Date	Population	Recommendations	Comments	Source
Stroke (continued)	AHA	2001	Hyperlipidemia	See screening recommendations on page 34. AHA endorses the NCEP II guidelines for management of hyperlipidemia (see algorithm in page 132)		Circulation 2001;103:163.
	AHA	2001	Smoking	Strongly encourage patient and family to stop smoking. Provide counseling, nicotine replacement, and formal programs as available.		Circulation 2001;103:163.

[a] Atrial fibrillation risk factors: hypertension, diabetes mellitus, poor left ventricular function, rheumatic mitral valve disease, prior TIA/stroke, systemic embolism or stroke, prosthetic heart valve (may require higher target INR).

[b] Risk factors for subsequent stroke in patients with atrial fibrillation include previous transient ischemic attack or stroke, hypertension, diabetes, thyrotoxicosis, mitral stenosis, or other forms of heart disease.

3
Disease Management

ADULT PATIENT WITH ALLERGIC RHINITIS: DIAGNOSIS AND MANAGEMENT
Source: American Academy of Allergy, Asthma and Immunology (AAAAI; and American College of Allergy, Asthma and Immunology (ACAAI)

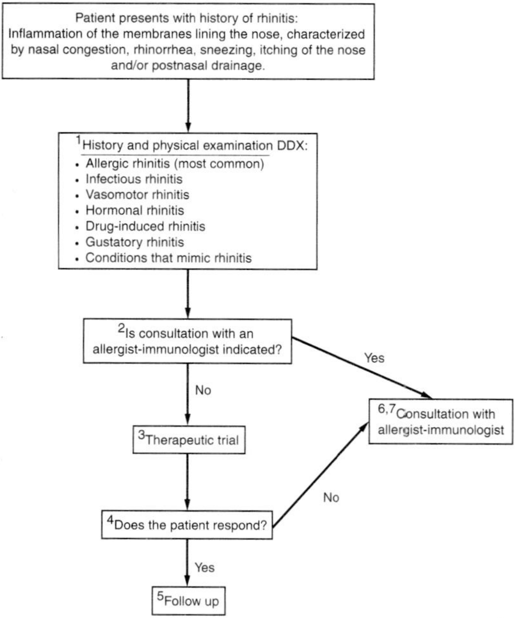

Adapted from: Diagnosis and Management of Rhinitis: Parameter Documents of the Joint Task Force on Practice Parameters in Allergy, Asthma and Immunology. American Academy of Allergy, Asthma and Immunology (AAAAI) and American College of Allergy, Asthma and Immunology (ACAAI). 1998. (http://www.jcaai.org)

Adult Rhinitis Algorithm: Notes

1. History: (a) presenting symptoms (eg, rhinorrhea, nasal congestion, sneezing, ocular sx); (b) length of symptomatology; (c) past medications taken for rhinitis, their effectiveness and adverse effects; (d) other medications; (e) degree to which rhinitis sx interfere with patient's ability to function and affect patient's quality of life; (f) seasonality and known triggers; (g) other medical conditions; (h) complications (eg, otitis media); (i) associated comorbid conditions (eg, asthma). Physical exam: (a) evaluation of nose—appearance of nasal mucous membranes, patency of nasal passageways, quality and quantity of nasal discharge; (b) evaluation of ears, eyes, throat and lungs.
2. Consider initial referral if: (a) need to define allergic/environmental triggers of rhinitis sx; (b) need for more intense education; (c) requires multiple medications over a prolonged period of time.
3. (a) **Avoidance of inciting factors.**
   (b) **Oral antihistamines:** Effective in reducing symptoms of itching, sneezing, and rhinorrhea. First line therapy for treatment of allergic rhinitis. Little objective effect on nasal congestion. Second generation antihistamines that are associated with less risk or no risk for sedation and performance impairment should usually be considered before sedating antihistamines.
   (c) **Intranasal antihistamines:** Appropriate first line treatment. May help reduce nasal congestion. Sedation may occur from systemic absorption.
   (d) **Oral decongestants:** Can effectively reduce nasal congestion. Can cause insomnia, anorexia, excessive nervousness. May increase BP.
   (e) **Nasally inhaled steroids:** Most effective medication class for controlling sx of allergic rhinitis. May be considered for initial tx without a prior trial of antihistamines and/or oral decongestants, and should be considered before initiating tx with systemic corticosteroids.
   (f) **Oral corticosteroids:** Should be reserved for severe cases of rhinitis. Short burst (5–7 days) preferred over depot parenteral corticosteroids which should be avoided.
   (g) **Intranasal cromolyn sodium:** Can reduce sx of allergic rhinitis in some patients; is most likely effective if initiated before sx become severe.
   (h) **Intranasal anticholinergics:** May effectively reduce rhinorrhea but have no effect on other nasal sx.
4. Assessing response to therapy: nasal symptoms, physical signs of rhinitis, quality of life. Include assessment of concomitant conditions (eg, asthma). If no good response to treatment, consider referral to allergist-immunologist. Reasons for referral: (a) duration of rhinitis sx > 3 months; (b) complications of rhinitis (eg, otitis media, sinusitis, nasal polyps); (c) comorbid conditions (eg, asthma); (d) requires oral corticosteroids for rhinitis; (e) symptoms interfere with patient's ability to function; (f) symptoms significantly decrease patient's quality of life; (g) treatment with medications for rhinitis are ineffective or produce adverse events; (h) need to define allergic/environmental triggers of rhinitis sx; (i) need for more intense education; (j) requires multiple medications over a prolonged period of time.
5. If initial tx successful, follow patient to assure continued control of sx, maintenance of improved quality of life, absence of medication side effects and reinforce education.
6. Includes detailed hx and physical examination. Additional examination may include: rhinoscopy, immediate hypersensitivity skin tests or in vitro tests to confirm an underlying allergic basis for symptoms. Nasal cytology may differentiate allergic rhinitis from other forms of rhinitis (eosinophils may indicate allergic rhinitis; neutrophils may support a dx of infectious rhinosinusitis). There is lack of expert consensus about whether nasal cytology should routinely be performed in the evaluation of rhinitis.

Neither total serum IgE nor total circulating eosinophil counts are routinely indicated as they are neither sensitive nor specific for allergic rhinitis. Specific tests may be necessary for co-existing conditions (eg, asthma, nasal polyps, sinusitis).

7. Specific immunotherapy (SIT) should be considered if: pharmacotherapy insufficiently controls sx or produces undesirable side effects; appropriate avoidance measures of indoor allergens fails to control sx; hx of allergic rhinitis for at least 2 seasons (seasonal) or 6 months (perennial); positive skin test results or serum-specific IgE that correlates with rhinitis sx. (American Academy of Otolaryngic Allergy [AAOA]. Allergic rhinitis: clinical practice guideline. Otolaryngol Head Neck Surg 1996;115[1]:115–22)

MANAGEMENT OF OSTEOARTHRITIS OF HIP AND KNEE
Source: American College of Rheumatology

Step-1

Non-Pharmacologic Therapy

- Patient education
- Self-management programs
- Personalized social support through telephone contact
- Weight loss (if overweight)
- Aerobic exercise programs
- Physical therapy
  - Range-of-motion
  - Muscle-strengthening (1)
- Assistive devices for ambulation
- Patellar taping
- Appropriate footwear
- Lateral-wedged insoles (for genu varum)
- Occupational therapy
  - Joint protection
  - Activities of daily living

↓ ***inadequate symptom relief***

Step-2

Acetaminophen (2) (total daily does not to exceed 4.0 gm/day)
*If moderate-to-severe **inflammation present**, consider **NSAID first (3)**.*

↓ ***inadequate symptom relief***

Step-3

Evaluate Renal and Gastrointestinal Risk

Renal Risk Present?
creatinine ≥ 2.0 mg/dL
\+
(1 of the following)
age ≥ 65 yrs, hypertension, congestive heart failure, OR diuretic or ACE inhibitor therapy

Yes →

Treatment Options

Non-NSAID Oral Therapy
- *Tramadol*
- *Salsalate*

Intra-articular therapy
- *Glucocorticoids*
- *Hyaluronan (4)*

Topical therapy (5)
- *Capsaicin*
- *Methylsalicylate*

↓ ***No***

GI Risk Present?
(at least 1 of the following)
age ≥ 65 yrs
comorbidity
oral glucocorticoid Rx
peptic ulcer disease Hx
upper GI bleed Hx
anticoagulant Rx

Yes →

Intra-articular therapy
- *Glucocorticoids*
- *Hyaluronan (4)*

Topical therapy (5)
- *Capsaicin*
- *Methylsalicylate*

Oral Therapy
- *Salsalate*
- *COX-2 inhibitors (6)*
- *NSAID + misoprostol or proton pump inhibitor*
- *Tramadol*

No →

Oral Therapy
- *Non-selective NSAID, or other therapies above (7)*

↓ ***inadequate symptom relief***

Step-4

Consider additional or alternative therapies
- **Opioid therapy**
- **Total joint arthroplasty (8)**

Adapted from: American College of Rheumatology Subcommittee on Osteoarthritis Guidelines. Recommendations for the Medical Management of Osteoarthritis of the Hip and Knee. Arthritis and Rheumatism 2000; 43:1905–15.

FOOTNOTES

1. Quadriceps weakness may precede, initiate and exacerbate knee osteoarthritis. (Rheum Dis Clin North Am 1999;25:283–98).
2. For many patients with mild-moderate osteoarthritis, pain relief with acetaminophen is comparable to NSAID. (Semin Arthritis Rheum 1997;27:755–70)
3. NSAIDs appear to be superior to acetaminophen in patients with severe pain related to osteoarthritis. (Arthritis Rheum 2000;43:378–85; J Rheumatol 2000;27:1020–7)
4. Hyaluronan intraarticular therapy has only been evaluated in knee osteoarthritis.
5. Topical therapy primarily indicated for mild-to-moderate pain related to osteoarthritis of the knee. There are no studies of topical therapy for hip osteoarthritis.
6. COX-2 inhibitors (celecoxib and rofecoxib) are as efficacious as non-selective NSAIDs, but not more efficacious. In contrast to non-selective NSAIDs, COX-2 inhibitors do not impair platelet function or bleeding time.
7. Use of concomitant gastroprotective therapy with misoprostol or a proton pump inhibitor is not recommended in the low risk patient.
8. No well-controlled trials of arthroscopic debridement with or without arthroplasty have been conducted. However, total joint arthroplasty provides marked pain relief and functional improvement in the vast majority of patients with osteoarthritis, and has been shown to be cost-effective in selected patients. An NIH Consensus conference recommends total hip replacement when "radiographic evidence of joint damage and moderate-to-severe persistent pain and disability, or both, that is not substantially relieved by an extended course of non-surgical management" is present.

ASTHMA: EVALUATION & MANAGEMENT

STEPWISE APPROACH FOR MANAGING ASTHMA IN ADULTS AND CHILDREN OLDER THAN 5 YEARS OF AGE

GOALS OF ASTHMA TREATMENT

Prevent, chronic and troublesome symptoms (eg, coughing or breathlessness in the night, in the early morning, or after exertion).
Maintain (near) "normal" pulmonary function.
Maintain normal activity levels (including exercise and other physical activity).
Prevent recurrent exacerbations of asthma and minimize the need for emergency department visits or hospitalizations.
Provide optimal pharmacotherapy with minimal or no adverse effects.
Meet patients' and families' expectations of and satisfaction with asthma care.

Classify Severity of Asthma

	Clinical Features before Treatment[a]		
	Symptoms[b]	**Nighttime Symptoms**	**Lung Function**
STEP 4 Severe Persistent	Continual symptoms Limited physical activity Frequent exacerbations	Frequent	FEV1 or PEF < 60% predicted PEF variability > 30%
STEP 3 Moderate Persistent	Daily symptoms Daily use of inhaled short-acting $beta_2$- agonist Exacerbations affect activity Exacerbations = 2 times a week; may last days	> 1 time a week	FEV1 or PEF > 60% – < 80% predicted PEF variability > 30%
STEP 2 Mild Persistent	Symptoms > 2 times a week but < 1 time a day Exacerbations may affect activity	> 2 times a month	FEV1 or PEF = 80% predicted PEF variability 20–30%

STEPWISE APPROACH FOR MANAGING ASTHMA IN ADULTS AND CHILDREN OLDER THAN 5 YEARS OF AGE (CONTINUED)

Classify Severity of Asthma			
	Clinical Features before Treatment[a]		
	Symptoms[b]	**Nighttime Symptoms**	**Lung Function**
STEP 1 Mild Intermittent	Symptoms ≤2 times a week Asymptomatic and normal PEF between exacerbations Exacerbations brief (from a few hours to a few days); intensity may vary	≤2 times a month	FEV1 or PEF = 80% predicted PEF variability < 20%

[a]The presence of one of the features of severity is sufficient to place a patient in that category. An individual should be assigned to the most severe grade in which any feature occurs. The characteristics noted in this table are general and may overlap because asthma is highly variable. Furthermore, an individual's classification may change over time.

[b]Patients at any level of severity can have mild, moderate, or severe exacerbations. Some patients with intermittent asthma experience severe and life-threatening exacerbations separated by long periods of normal lung function and no symptoms. FEV1 = forced expiratory volume in 1 second; PEF = peak expiratory flow.

Source: National Heart, Lung and Blood Institute; NIH. http://www.nhlbi.gov/guidelines/asthma/asthgdln.htm

ASTHMA: EVALUATION & MANAGEMENT

STEPWISE APPROACH FOR MANAGING ASTHMA IN ADULTS AND CHILDREN OLDER THAN 5 YEARS OF AGE: TREATMENT

	Long-Term Control	Quick Relief	Education
STEP 4 Severe Persistent	Daily medications: Anti-inflammatory: inhaled corticosteroid (high dose) AND Long-acting bronchodilator: either long-acting inhaled $beta_2$-agonist, sustained-release theophylline, or long-acting $beta_2$-agonist tablets AND Corticosteroid tablets or syrup long term (make repeat attempts to reduce systemic steroids and maintain control with high-dose inhaled steroids)	Short-acting bronchodilator: inhaled $beta_2$-agonists as needed for symptoms Intensity of treatment will depend on severity of exacerbation. Use of short-acting inhaled $beta_2$-agonists on a daily basis, or increasing use, indicates the need for additional long-term-control therapy.	Steps 2 and 3 actions plus: Refer to individual education/counseling.

STEPWISE APPROACH FOR MANAGING ASTHMA IN ADULTS AND CHILDREN OLDER THAN 5 YEARS OF AGE: TREATMENT (CONTINUED)

	Long-Term Control	**Quick Relief**	**Education**
STEP 3 Moderate Persistent	Daily medication: Either Anti-inflammatory: inhaled corticosteroid (medium dose) OR Inhaled corticosteroid (low-medium dose) and add a long-acting bronchodilator, especially for nighttime symptoms; either long-acting inhaled beta$_2$-agonist, sustained-release theophylline, or long-acting beta$_2$-agonist tablets If needed; Anti-inflammatory: inhaled corticosteroids (medium-high dose) AND Long-acting bronchodilator, especially for nighttime symptoms: either long-acting inhaled beta$_2$-agonist, sustained-release theophylline, or long-acting beta$_2$-agonist tablets	Short-acting bronchodilator: inhaled beta$_2$-agonists as needed for symptoms Intensity of treatment will depend on severity of exacerbation. Use of short-acting inhaled beta$_2$-agonists on a daily basis, or increasing use, indicates the need for additional long-term-control therapy.	Step 1 actions plus: Teach self-monitoring. Refer to group education if available. Review and update self-management plan.

STEPWISE APPROACH FOR MANAGING ASTHMA IN ADULTS AND CHILDREN OLDER THAN 5 YEARS OF AGE: TREATMENT (CONTINUED)

	Long-Term Control	Quick Relief	Education
STEP 2 Mild Persistent	One daily medication: Anti-inflammatory: either inhaled corticosteroid (low doses) or cromolyn or nedocromil (children usually begin with a trial of cromolyn or nedocromil) Sustained-release theophylline to serum concentration of 5–15 mg/L is an alternative, but not preferred, therapy. Zafirlukast or zileuton may also be considered for patients > 12 years of age, although their position in therapy is not fully established.	Short-acting bronchodilator: inhaled beta$_2$-agonists as needed for symptoms Intensity of treatment will depend on severity of exacerbation. Use of short-acting inhaled beta$_2$-agonists on a daily basis, or increasing use, indicates the need for additional long-term-control therapy.	Step 1 actions plus: Teach self-monitoring. Refer to group education if available. Review and update self-management plan.

ASTHMA: EVALUATION & MANAGEMENT

STEPWISE APPROACH FOR MANAGING ASTHMA IN ADULTS AND CHILDREN OLDER THAN 5 YEARS OF AGE: TREATMENT (CONTINUED)

	Long-Term Control	Quick Relief	Education
STEP 1 Mild Intermittent	No daily medication needed	Short-acting bronchodilator: inhaled beta$_2$-agonists as needed for symptoms Intensity of treatment will depend on severity of exacerbation. Use of short-acting inhaled beta$_2$-agonists more than 2 times a week may indicate the need to initiate long-term-control therapy.	Teach basic facts about asthma. Teach inhaler/spacer/holding chamber technique. Discuss roles of medications. Develop self-management plan. Develop action plan for when and how to take rescue actions, especially for patients with a history of severe exacerbations. Discuss appropriate environmental control measures to avoid exposure to known allergens and irritants.

STEPWISE APPROACH FOR MANAGING ASTHMA IN ADULTS AND CHILDREN OLDER THAN 5 YEARS OF AGE: TREATMENT (CONTINUED)	
Step down: Review treatment every 16 months; a gradual stepwise reduction in treatment may be possible.	Step up: If control is not maintained, consider step up. First, review patient medication technique, adherence, and environmental control (avoidance of allergens or other factors that contribute to asthma severity).

Note: The stepwise approach presents general guidelines to assist clinical decision making; it is not intended to be a specific prescription. Asthma is highly variable; clinicians should tailor specific medication plans to the needs and circumstances of individual patients.

Gain control as quickly as possible; then decrease treatment to the least medication necessary to maintain control. Gaining control may be accomplished by either starting treatment at the step most appropriate to the initial severity of the condition or starting at a higher level or therapy (eg, a course of systemic corticosteroids or higher dose of inhaled corticosteroids).

A rescue course of systemic corticosteroids may be needed at any time and at any step.

Some patients with intermittent asthma experience severe and life-threatening exacerbations separated by long periods of normal lung function and no symptoms. This may be especially common with exacerbations provoked by respiratory infections. A short course of systemic corticosteroids is recommended.

At each step, patients should control their environment to avoid or control factors that make their asthma worse (eg, allergens, irritants); this requires specific diagnosis and education.

Referral to an asthma specialist for consultation or co-management is recommended if there are difficulties achieving or maintaining control of asthma or if the patient requires step 4 care. Referral may be considered if the patient requires step 3 care.

Source: National Heart, Lung and Blood Institute; NIH. http://www.nhlbi.nih.gov/guidelines/asthma/asthgdln.htm

ATOPIC DERMATITIS: EVALUATION & MANAGEMENT ALGORITHM
Source: American College of Allergy, Asthma and Immunology

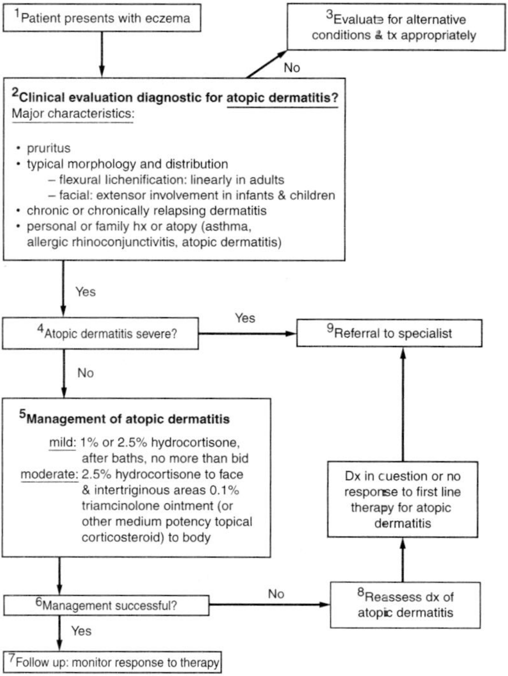

Adapted from: Disease Management of Atopic Dermatitis: A Practice Parameter. Am Allergy Asthma Immunol 1997 Sep; 79(3):197–211. (http://www.jcaai.org)

Atopic Dermatitis: Evaluation and Management Algorithm Notes

1. **Eczema** refers to a pruritic dermatitis that includes a long list of differential diagnoses (see notes 2 and 3).
2. **Other characteristics of atopic dermatitis** (in the absence of an atopic history, 3 or more required for diagnosis): xerosis; ichthyosis/palmar hyperlinearity/keratosis pilaris; immediate, Type I skin test response; hand and/or foot dermatitis; cheilitis; nipple eczema; susceptibility to cutaneous infections; erythroderma; early age of onset; impaired cell-mediated immunity; recurrent conjunctivitis; infraorbital fold; keratoconus; anterior subscapular cataracts; elevated total serum IgE; peripheral blood eosinophils. **History:** pruritic nature of rash, age of onset, duration, triggers, seasonal variation, eye complications, environmental exposures, chronicity, distribution of rash. **Physical examination:** morphology and distribution of the atopic skin lesions, especially noting diffuse xerosis, erythema, excoriation, papulation, crusting/oozing/ pustules indicative of infection, scaling, lichenification. Look for associated characteristics. **Laboratory testing:** skin or in vitro testing for specific allergens. The majority of patients have elevated serum IgE and eosinophilia; these findings are not useful in guiding clinical decisions. A diagnosis of atopic dermatitis cannot be made solely on the basis of laboratory testing.
3. **Differential diagnosis of atopic dermatitis**
   - Immunodeficiencies: Wiskott-Aldrich syndrome, DiGeorge syndrome, Hyper-IgE syndrome, severe combined immune deficiency
   - Metabolic diseases: Phenylketonuria, tyrosinemia, histidinemia, multiple carboxylase deficiency, essential fatty acid deficiency
   - Neoplastic disease: Cutaneous T-cell lymphoma, histiocytosis X, Sézary syndrome
   - Infection and infestation: Candida, herpes simplex, *Staphylococcus aureus*, *Sarcoptes scabiei*
   - Dermatitis: Contact, seborrheic, psoriasis
4. **Severe atopic dermatitis:**
   - More than 20% skin involvement (or 10% skin involvement if affected areas include the eyelids, hands or intertriginous areas)
   - Extensive skin involvement and erythrodermic, at risk for exfoliation
   - Requiring ongoing or frequent treatment with high potency topical glucocorticoids or systemic glucocorticoids
   - Requiring hospitalization for severe eczema or skin infections related to atopic dermatitis
   - Ocular or infectious complications
   - Significant disruption of quality of life
5. Treatment of atopic dermatitis is directed at symptom relief and reduction of cutaneous inflammation. Characterization of each patient's atopic dermatitis severity and reduction of exacerbating factors are critical for effective management. All patients require skin hydration in combination with an effective emollient. Potential trigger factors should be identified and eliminated.
6. Response to therapy is classified as complete response, partial response, or treatment failure. Since atopic dermatitis is a chronic relapsing skin condition, most patients will have a partial response with reduction in pruritus and extent of skin disease.

7. Follow-up is required to monitor the patient's response to therapy and adjust medications and skin care according to severity of illness. A plan should be established to step-up medications for flare-ups and to step-down medications when the illness is under control.
8. In any patient who fails to respond to treatment, it is important to reassess the diagnosis to be certain the patient has atopic dermatitis. In patients presenting after the age of 16 years, consider contact dermatitis. In patients presenting as adults, consider cutaneous T cell lymphoma.
9. The patient who does not respond to first line therapy, or who has severe atopic dermatitis (note 4) is highly challenging and requires a multidisciplinary approach that may exceed the resources of the primary care physician. For these patients, consultation with a specialist who is skilled in the management of patients with severe atopic dermatitis can be beneficial.

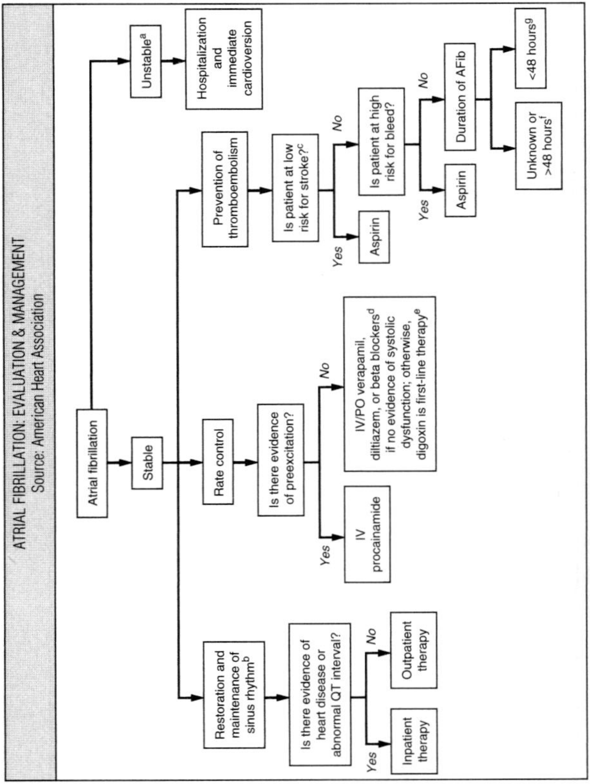

ATRIAL FIBRILLATION: EVALUATION & MANAGEMENT
Source: American Heart Association

ATRIAL FIBRILLATION: EVALUATION & MANAGEMENT (CONTINUED)
Source: American Heart Association

[a] Evidence of Wolff-Parkinson-White syndrome or pre-excitation, hypotension, or congestive heart failure.

[b] Maintenance of sinus rhythm after cardioversion is improved by treatment with quinidine, procainamide, disopyramide, propafenone, sotalol, flecainide, or amiodarone. Selection of an antiarrhythmic agent should take into account the patient's liver and renal function, comorbidities, and systolic function.

[c] Patients at high stroke risk (thromboembolic rates > 5% per year) include those with a history of hypertension, prior stroke/transient ischemic attack, diabetes, age > 65 years, impaired systolic function, and enlarged left atrial size. Low-risk patients have a thromboembolic risk of 1—1.5% per year. (Arch Intern Med 1994;154:1449; Ann Intern Med 1992;116:1).

[d] Beta-blockers are especially effective in the setting of thyrotoxicosis or increased sympathetic tone (eg, alcohol withdrawal).

[e] If rate is difficult to control with pharmacologic therapy, consider AV node ablation or modification.

[f] Two options: (1) Anticoagulate x 3 weeks (INR 2.0—3.0), followed by electrical/pharmacologic cardioversion; if successful, continue anticoagulation for an additional 4 weeks; or (2) begin IV heparin and perform transesophageal echocardiography; if no atrial thrombus, then perform cardioversion followed by 4 weeks of anticoagulation. Patients age > 75 years should be monitored more closely for therapeutic INR and perhaps be kept closer to 2.0.

[g] Cardioversion can be performed. There are few data to guide the need for anticoagulation.

AFib = atrial fibrilllation

Source: Adapted form AHA Subcommittee on Electrocardiography and Electrophysiology, Circulation 1996;93:1262.

CATARACT IN ADULTS: EVALUATION & MANAGEMENT ALGORITHM
Source: Agency for Healthcare Research and Quality

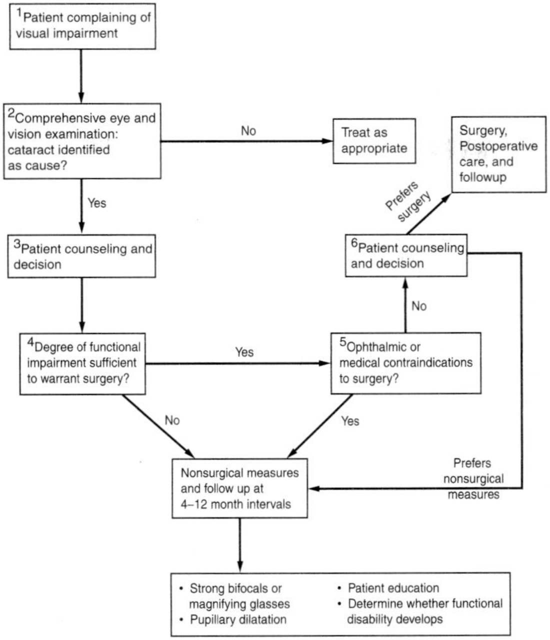

Adapted from: Cataract in Adults: Management of Functional Impairment (Clinical Practice Guideline). Publication No. AHCPR 93-0542. Rockville, MD: Agency for Health Care Research and Quality Public Health Service, US Department of Health and Human Services, February, 1993.

Cataract in Adults: Evaluation & Management Algorithm, Notes

1. Cataract evaluation and management should begin only when patients complain of a visual problem or impairment. Identifying impairment in visual function during routine history and physical examination constitutes sound medical practice.
2. Essential elements of the comprehensive eye and vision examination:
   - Patient history. Consider cataracts if: acute or gradual onset of vision loss; vision problems under special conditions (eg, low contrast, glare); difficulties performing various visual tasks. Ask about: refractive history; previous ocular disease; amblyopia; eye surgery; trauma; general health history; medications; and allergies. In addition, it is critical to describe the actual impact of the cataract on the person's function and quality of life. There are several instruments available for assessing functional impairment related to cataract, including VF-14, Activities of Daily Vision Scale, and Visual Activities Questionnaire.
   - Ocular examination, including: Snellen acuity and refraction; measurement of intraocular pressure; assessment of pupillary function; external examination; slit-lamp examination; and dilated examination of fundus.
   - Supplemental testing: May be necessary to assess and document the extent of the functional disability and to determine whether other diseases may limit preoperative or postoperative vision.

   Most elderly patients presenting with visual problems do not have a cataract that causes functional impairment. Refractive error, macular degeneration, and glaucoma are common alternative etiologies for visual impairment.
3. Once cataract has been identified as the cause of visual disability, patients should be counseled concerning the nature of the problem, its natural history, and the existence of both surgical and nonsurgical approaches to management. The principal factor that should guide decision making with regard to surgery is the extent to which the cataract impairs the ability to function in daily life. The findings of the physical examination should corroborate that the cataract is the major contributing cause of the functional impairment, and that there is a reasonable expectation that managing the cataract will positively impact the patient's functional activity. Visual acuity is not the *sole* determining factor, and should not be used as a threshold value.
4. Patients who complain of mild to moderate limitation in activities due to a visual problem, those whose corrected acuities are near 20/40, and those who do not yet wish to undergo surgery may be offered nonsurgical measures for improving visual function. Indications for surgery: cataract-impaired vision no longer meets the patient's needs; evidence of lens-induced disease (eg, phakomorphic glaucoma, phakolytic glaucoma); necessary to visualize the fundus in an eye that has the potential for sight (eg, diabetic patient who is at risk of diabetic nephropathy).
5. Contraindications to surgery: the patient does not desire surgery; glasses or visual aids provide satisfactory functional vision; surgery will not improve visual function; the patient's quality of life is not compromised; the patient is unable to undergo surgery because of coexisting medical or ocular conditions; a legal consent cannot be obtained; or the patient is unable to obtain adequate postoperative care. Routine preoperative medical testing (12-lead EKG, CBC, measurement of serum electrolytes, BUN, creatinine, and glucose), while commonly performed in patients scheduled to undergo cataract surgery, does not appear to measurably increase the safety of the surgery.
6. Patients with significant functional and visual impairment due to cataract who have no contraindications to surgery should be counseled regarding the expected risks and benefits of surgery and alternatives to surgery.

Sources

American Academy of Ophthalmology and American Society of Cataract and Refractive Surgery. White Paper on Cataract Surgery. (http://www.ascrs.org/eye/white.html, accessed 1/28/01).

American Optometric Association Consensus Panel on Care of the Adult Patient with Cataract. Optometric Clinical Practice Guideline: Care of the Adult Patient with Cataract. Updated 3/30/99. (http://www.aoanet.org, site accessed 1/28/01).

Cataract in the Adult Eye. American Academy of Ophthalmology (AAO). 1996. PO Box 7424, San Francisco, CA 94120-7424, (415) 561-8540, www.eyenet.org.

Cataract Management Guideline Panel. Cataract in Adults: Management of Functional Impairment. Clinical Practice Guideline, Number 4, Rockville, MD. US Department of Health and Human Services, Agency for Health Care Policy and Research. AHCPR Pub. No. 93-0542. Feb. 1993.

Mangione CM, Phillips RS, Seddon JM, Lawrence MG, Cook EF, Dailey R, Goldman L. Development of the Activities of Daily Vision Scale—A Measure of Visual Functional Status. Medical Care 1992;30: 1111–1126.

Schein OD, Katz J, Bass EB, Tielsch JM, Lubomski LH, Feldman MA, Petty PG, Steinberg EP. The value of routine preoperative medical testing before cataract surgery. N Engl J Med 2000;342:168–75.

Sloane ME, Ball K, Owsley C, Bruni JR, Roenker DL. The Visual Activities Questionnaire: Developing an instrument for assessing problems in everyday visual tasks. Technical Digest, Noninvasive Assessment of the Visual System. 1992;1:26–29.

Steinberg EP, Tielsch JM, Schein OD, Javitt JC, Sharkey P, Cassard SC, Legro MW, Diener-West M, Bass EB, Damiano AM, Steinwachs D, Simmer A. The VF-14. An index of functional impairment in patients with cataract. Arch Ophthalmol 112;994:630–638.

CERVICAL PAP SMEAR ABNORMALITIES: MANAGEMENT AND FOLLOW-UP[a]

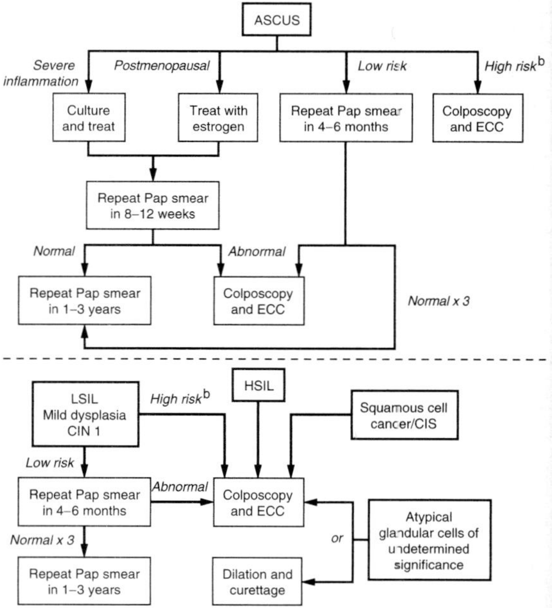

[a]Assumes satisfactory specimen; if unsatisfactory, repeat Pap smear.
[b]High risk = any history of abnormal Pap smear, poor compliance, unlikely to return for follow-up, any human papillomavirus (HPV) changes.
ASCUS = atypical squamous cells of undetermined significance; ECC = endocervical curettage; LSIL = low-grade squamous intraepithelial lesion; CIN = cervical intraepithelial neoplasia; HSIL = high-grade squamous intraepithelial lesion; CIS = carcinoma in situ.
Source: Modified from Rosenfeld JA (editor): Women s Health in Primary Care. Williams & Wilkins, 1997.

EVALUATING THE ADULT WITH ACUTE, NON-TRAUMATIC CHEST PAIN: RECOMMENDED ACTIONS IN RESPONSE TO IMPORTANT HISTORICAL ELEMENTS

	Actions									
Character of Pain	**A**	**B**	**C**	**D**	**E**	**F**	**G**	**H**	**I**	**J**
1. Ongoing **and** severe **and** crushing **and** substernal **or** same as previous MI pain	++	++	+					+		
2. Severe or pressure or substernal or exertional or radiating to jaw, neck shoulder or arm	++	+	+					+		
3. Tearing, severe, and radiating to the back	++	++	++	+						
4. Similar to that of previous pulmonary embolus	++	++	+		++				+	
5. Indigestion or burning epigastric	+									
6. Pleuritic	+		+							
Patient Age										
7. Male > 33 years; Female > 40 years	+									
Associated Symptoms										
8. Syncope or near syncope	++	+								3
9. SOB, DOE, PND, or orthopnea	++		+						+	
10. Significant hemoptysis			++						+	
11. Nausea/vomiting	+									
12. Productive or chronic cough										
13. Palpitations	+	+								
14. Significant weight change			+							
15. Diaphoresis	+									
Past Medical History										
16. Previous MI	++									
17. Coronary artery bypass graft/angioplasty	++									
18. Cocaine use within last 96 hours	++									1

EVALUATING THE ADULT WITH ACUTE, NON-TRAUMATIC CHEST PAIN: RECOMMENDED ACTIONS IN RESPONSE TO IMPORTANT HISTORICAL ELEMENTS (CONTINUED)										
	Actions									
Past Medical History (continued)	**A**	**B**	**C**	**D**	**E**	**F**	**G**	**H**	**I**	**J**
19. Previous positive cardiac diagnostic studies	++									2
20. Cardiac medications (current)	+									1
21. Diuretics (current)										2
22. IV drug use (current)	+		+						+	
23. Major risk factors for coronary artery disease (a)	+									
24. Major risk factors for pulmonary embolus (b)	+		+		+	+			+	
25. Major risk factors for thoracic aortic aneurysm/dissection (c)	+		+	+						
26. Major risk factors for pericarditis/myocarditis (d)	+		+				+	+		
27. Major risk factors for pneumothorax (e)			+							
28. Major risk factors for pneumonia (f)			+						+	

EVALUATING THE ADULT WITH ACUTE, NON-TRAUMATIC CHEST PAIN: RECOMMENDED ACTIONS IN RESPONSE TO IMPORTANT HISTORICAL ELEMENTS (CONTINUED)

A = ECG; B = cardiac monitor; C = CXR; D = aortic imaging; E = pulmonary vasculature imaging; F = venous imaging; G = echocardiography; H = cardiac serum markers; I = ABG and/or oximetry; J = other testing (see footnotes).

(a) Coronary artery disease risk factors include: family hx; men age > 45 yrs, women age > 55 yrs; diabetes; hypertension; cigarette use; left ventricular hypertrophy; elevated cholesterol levels; hx chronic cocaine use.
(b) Pulmonary embolus risk factors include: prolonged immobilization; surgery > 30 min within past 3 months; hx DVT or pulmonary embolus; malignancy; pregnancy or recent pregnancy; hx of pelvis or lower extremity trauma; oral contraceptive use plus cigarette use; CHF; COPD; obesity; hypercoagulable state
(c) Thoracic aortic aneurysm/dissection risk factors include: hypertension; congenital disease of aorta or aortic valve; inflammatory disease of the aorta; connective tissue disease; pregnancy; arteriosclerosis; cigarette use.
(d) Pericarditis/myocarditis risk factors include: infections (eg, tuberculosis, viral); autoimmune/systematic disease (eg, lupus); acute rheumatic fever; recent MI or cardiac surgery; malignancy; radiation therapy to mediastinum; uremia; drugs (procainamide, hydralazine, INH, etc); hx of prior pericarditis
(e) Pneumothorax risk factors include: hx of previous pneumothorax; Valsalva maneuver; lung disease (obstructive, cancer, infection, connective tissue disease); cigarette use
(f) Pneumonia risk factors include: chronic lung disease; altered consciousness/impaired gag reflex; neuromuscular disease; thoracic cage deformity; cigarette use; preceding viral respiratory infection; immunodeficiency

1. Measurement of appropriate serum drug levels should be considered.
2. Measurement of K+ and Mg++ serum levels should be considered.
3. Measurement of the hematocrit should be considered.

Modified from: American College of Emergency Physicians: Clinical policy for the initial approach to adults presenting with a chief complaint of chest pain, with no history of trauma. Ann Emerg Med 1995; 25:274–299

EVALUATING THE ADULT WITH ACUTE, NON-TRAUMATIC CHEST PAIN: RECOMMENDED ACTIONS IN RESPONSE TO IMPORTANT PHYSICAL EXAMINATION FINDINGS

	Actions									
Vital Signs	**A**	**B**	**C**	**D**	**E**	**F**	**G**	**H**	**I**	**J**
1. Irregular pulse	+	++								
2. Tachypnea (RR > 24)	+								+	
3. Fever (> 38°C/100.4°F)			+							
4. Hypertension (SBP > 160 and/or DBP > 110)	+		+							
5. Tachycardia (> 100)	+								+	
6. Bradycardia (< 60)	+									
Appearance										
7. Cyanosis with respiratory distress	++	++	++		+				++	4
8. Diaphoresis	++		+					+	+	
Cardiovascular Exam										
9. Significant differences in right and left arm blood pressures	++	+	++	+						
10. New murmur	++		+				+			
11. Pericardial rub	++		+				+	+		
12. Irregular rhythm	+	++								
13. Jugular venous distention	+		+							
14. Third heart sound	+		+							
Pulmonary Exam										
15. Unilateral diminished breath sounds			++						+	
16. Localized dullness to percussion			+							
17. Pleural rub	+		+						+	
18. Unilateral rales			+						+	
19. Bilateral rales	+		+						+	
20. Wheezing	+	++	+						+	5

EVALUATING THE ADULT WITH ACUTE, NON-TRAUMATIC CHEST PAIN: RECOMMENDED ACTIONS IN RESPONSE TO IMPORTANT PHYSICAL EXAMINATION FINDINGS (CONTINUED)

	Actions									
Extremities	**A**	**B**	**C**	**D**	**E**	**F**	**G**	**H**	**I**	**J**
21. Unilateral leg swelling, pain, tenderness, warmth, erythema	+		+		+	+			+	
22. Bilateral edema	+		+							

++: An action reflecting principles of good practice in most situations. There may be circumstances when a rule need not or cannot be followed; in these situations, it is advisable that deviation from the rule be justified in writing.

+: An action that may be considered, depending on the patient, the circumstances, or other factors. Thus, these actions are not always followed, and there is no implication that failure to follow a guideline is improper.

A = ECG; B = cardiac monitor; C = CXR; D = aortic imaging; E = pulmonary vasculature imaging; F = venous imaging; G = echocardiography; H = cardiac serum markers; I = ABG and/or oximetry; J = other testing (see footnotes).

4. Consider methemoglobin level and intubation.
5. Consider spirometry and bendrodilator therapy.

Modified from: American College of Emergency Physicians: Clinical policy for the initial approach to adults presenting with a chief complaint of chest pain, with no history of trauma. Ann Emerg Med 1995; 25:274–299

LIPID AND CHOLESTEROL MANAGEMENT

Source: NCEP III

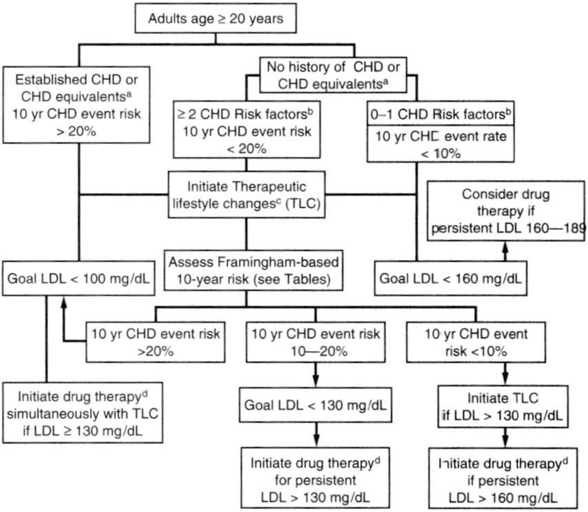

[a] CHD risk equivalents carry a risk for major coronary events equal to that of established CHD (ie, > 20% per 10 years), and include: diabetes, other clinical forms of arthrosclerotic disease (peripheral arterial disease, abdominal aortic aneurysm, and symptomatic carotid artery disease).

[b] Age (men ≥ 45 years, women ≥55 years or postmenopausal), hypertension (BP ≥ 140/90 mm Hg or on antihypertensive medication), cigarette smoking, HDL < 40 mg/dL, family history of premature CHD in first-degree relative (males < 55 years, females < 65 years). Diabetes now considered CHD risk equivalent. For HDL ≥ 60 mg/dL, subtract 1 risk factor from above.

[c] All patients, particularly those with elevated cholesterol levels, should be encouraged to adopt the following lifestyle changes: reduce saturated fat (< 7% total calories) and cholesterol (< 200 mg/d intake; increase physical activity; and achieve appropriate weight control (see publication for greater details on TLC regimens) assess affects of TLC on liquid levels after 3 months.

[d] Drug therapy response should be monitored and modified at 6 week intervals to acheve goal LDL levels after goal LDL met, monitor response and adhrenel every 4–6 months.

Source: Executive summary of the third report of the National Cholesterol Education Project (NCEP) expert panel on detection, evaluation and treatment of high blood cholesterol in adults (Adult Treatment Panel III). JAMA 2001;285:2486.

CHRONIC CONGESTIVE HEART FAILURE EVALUATION AND MANAGEMENT
Source: American Heart Association

DIAGNOSTIC STUDIES

Usually Indicated, Always Acceptable
- CBC, lytes, BUN, Cre, glucose, PO4, Mg,Ca, albumin
- urinalysis
- TSH
- chest Xray
- 12-lead ECG
- echocardiography
- cardiac stress test (1)
- cardiac catheterization (2)

Acceptable, Unproven Efficacy
- see footnote (#3)

Generally NOT Indicated
- Repeat coronary angiography or stress testing when coronary artery disease previously excluded and no objective evidence of intercurrent ischemia.
- Routine endomyocardial biopsy
- Multiple echocardiographic studies in the routine follow-up of patients with CHF responding to therapy.
- Routine Holter or signal-averaged ECG.
- Cardiac catheterization in patients who are not surgical candidates.

TREATMENT OF SYSTOLIC DYSFUNCTION

Usually Indicated, Always Acceptable
- ACE inhibitors (4)
- Diuretic agents, if fluid overload
- Digoxin (5)
- Beta-blockers for high-risk patients after acute MI

Acceptable, Unproven Efficacy
- see footnote #6

Generally NOT Indicated
- Calcium channel blockers in absence of coexistent angina/hypertension
- Treatment of asymptomatic ventricular rhythms

TREATMENT OF DIASTOLIC DYSFUNCTION

Usually Indicated, Always Acceptable
- Diuretic agents
- Nitrates

Acceptable, Unproven Efficacy
- see footnote #7

Generally NOT Indicated
- Positive inotropic drugs in absence of systolic dysfunction
- Treatment of asymptomatic arrhythmias

Acute Decompensations of Chronic Congestive Heart Failure

↓

Are Precipitating Factors of Concurrent Threatening Conditions Present (8)?

yes →
- See Acute Cardiogenic Pulmonary Edema Algorithm
- Hospitalization usually necessary

no → Assess Severity of Symptoms

- ***moderate-severe symptoms*** →
  - See Acute Cardiogenic Pulmonary Edema Algorithm
  - Hospitalization usually necessary
- ***mild-moderate symptoms*** →
  - Management in ER or outpatient facility

Adapted from: http://circ.ahajournals.org/cgi/content/full/92/9/2764
Hazinski MG, Cummins RD, Field JM (eds). 2000 Handbook of Emergency Cardiovascular Care for Healthcare Providers. American Heart Association, Dallas, TX, 2000. page 21. ISBN 0-87493-744-2

FOOTNOTES

1. If patient has coronary artery disease risk factors and no angina; or if patient has prior MI, no angina and is a revascularization candidate.
2. If (a) patient with angina or large areas of ischemic or hibernating myocardium; or (b) patient at risk for coronary artery disease who is undergoing surgical correction of non-coronary cardiac lesions.
3. (a) serum iron, ferritin; (b) stress testing, or (c) coronary arteriography in all patients with unexplained CHF who are candidates for revascularization; (d) endomycardial biopsy (unless recent onset of rapidly deteriorating cardiac function, suspected myocarditis, chemotherapy with myocardial toxic agents, or Hx of hemochromatosis, sarcoid, amyloid, Loeffler's endocarditis, or endomyocardial fibroelastosis).
4. Substitute hydralazine and isosorbide dinitrate in patients unable to tolerate ACE inhibitors.
5. Digoxin indicated when atrial fibrillation with rapid ventricular response present, or when patient is not adequately controlled with ACE inhibitor and diuretic therapy.
6. (a) digoxin for all patients; (b) addition of hydralazine and isosorbide dinitrate for patients not controlled with ACE inhibitor; (c) beta-blocker for dilated cardiomyopathy; (d) anticoagulation in patients with sinus rhythm and very low ejection fraction or intracardiac thrombus; and (e) outpatient low-dose dobutamine.
7. (a) calcium channel blockers; (b) beta-blockers; (c) ACE inhibitors; and (d) anticoagulation in patients with intracardiac thrombus.
8. Precipitating factors include recent MI; threatening conditions include marked hypokalemia, moderate-to-marked azotemia, and symptomatic arrhythmias.

DEPRESSION: MANAGEMENT

OVERVIEW OF TREATMENT FOR DEPRESSION
Source: Agency for Healthcare Research and Quality

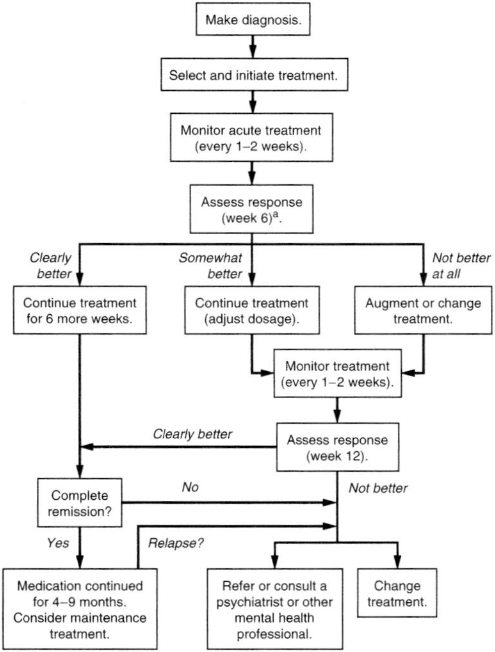

[a]Times of assessment (weeks 6 and 12) rest on very modest data. It may be necessary to revise the treatment plan earlier for patients who fail to respond at all.

Source: Reproduced, with permission, from Agency for Health Care Policy and Research: Depression in Primary Care. Vol. 2: Treatment of Major Depression. United States Department of Health and Human Services, 1993.

DIABETES MELLITUS: MANAGEMENT

MANAGEMENT OF HYPERGLYCEMIA[a]
Source: American Diabetes Association

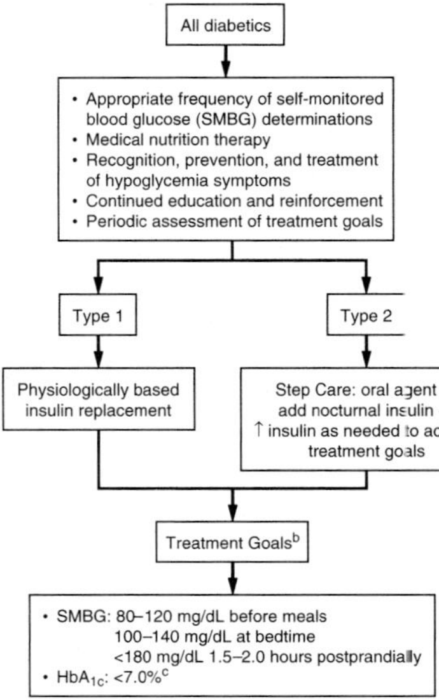

[a]Adapted from American Diabetes Association Position Statement Standards of Medical Care for Patients With Diabetes Mellitus. Last updated January 1999. (http://www.diabetes.org/DiabetesCare/Supplement199/S32.htm)

[b]These are generalized goals. They do not apply to pregnant adults. One should modify individual treatment goals to take into account risk for hypoglycemia, very young or old age, end-stage renal disease, advanced cardiovascular or cerebrovascular disease, or other diseases that decrease life expectancy.

[c]Based on results of the Diabetes Control and Complications Trial (DCCT) (Type 1) and the United Kingdom Prospective Diabetes Study (UKPDS) (Type 2).

DIABETES MELLITUS: PREVENTION AND TREATMENT OF COMPLICATIONS

PREVENTION & TREATMENT OF DIABETIC COMPLICATIONS

Complication	Goal	Monitoring	Action if Goal Not Met
Hyperglycemia	$HbA_{1c} < 7.0\%$	HbA_{1c} = every 6 months	See management, previous page
Retinopathy	Prevent vision loss	Annual retinal exam[a]	Laser treatment
Neuropathy	Prevent foot complications	Annual foot exam[b]	Examine feet at every visit
Nephropathy	Prevent renal failure	Annual urinary protein determination[c]	See below[d]
Hypertension	Adult: BP < 130/85 mm Hg Elderly: SBP < 160 mm Hg	Annual BP determination	Sec JNC VI, page 132
Hyperlipidemia	LDL < 100 mg/dL	Annual determination unless low risk	Weight loss; increase in physical activity; nutrition therapy; follow NCEP recommendations for pharmacologic treatment, Appendix VII

[a]Dilated eye exam or 7-field 30-degree fundus photography by ophthalmologist or optometrist.

[b]Includes evaluation of protective sensation, vascular status, and inspection for foot deformities or ulcers.

[c]Microalbuminuria treatment: if type 1: ACE inhibitor; if type 2: individualize decision. Clinical albuminuria treatment: (1) Achieve BP < 130/85 mm Hg; (2) use ACE inhibitor; (3) improve glycemic control; and (4) decrease protein to 10% of dietary intake. Refer to nephrologist if: glomerular filtration rate < 70 mL/min, creatinine > 2.0 mg/dL, or when management of hypertension or hyperkalemia is difficult.

Source: Adapted from American Diabetes Association Position Statement "Standards of Medical Care for Patients With Diabetes Mellitus." Last updated January 1999. (http://www.diabetes.org/DiabetesCare/Supplement199/S32.htm)

DIABETES MELLITUS: PREVENTION AND TREATMENT OF COMPLICATIONS

PREVENTION & TREATMENT OF DIABETIC COMPLICATIONS (CONTINUED)

Category	[c] Albuminuria Thresholds		
	24-h collection (mg/24 h)	Timed collection (μg/min)	Spot collection (μg/creatinine)
Normal	< 30	< 20	< 30
Microalbuminuria	30–300	20–200	30–300
Clinical albuminuria	> 300	> 200	> 300

Because of variability in urinary albumin excretion, two of three specimens collected within a 3- to 6-month period should be abnormal before considering a patient to have crossed one of these diagnostic thresholds. Exercise within 24 h, infection, fever, congestive heart failure, marked hyperglycemia, and marked hypertension may elevate urinary albumin excretion over baseline values.

HYPERTENSION: INITIATING THERAPY

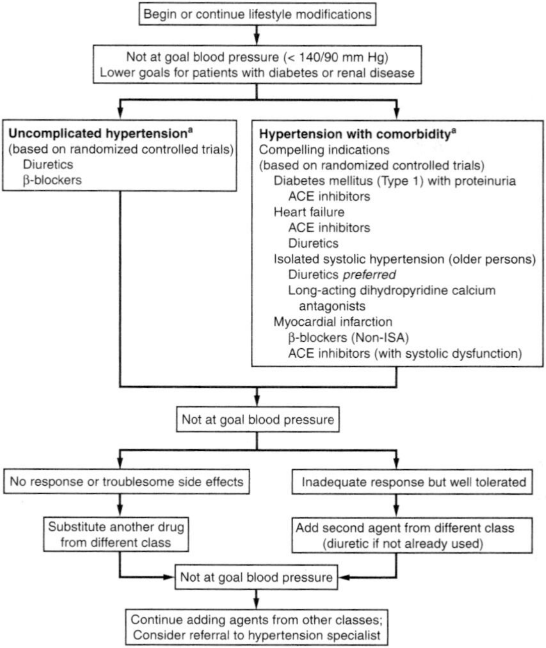

[a]Start with a low dose of a long-acting once-daily drug, and *titrate* dose. Low-dose combinations may be appropriate.

ACE = angiotensin-converting enzyme; ISA = intrinsic sympathomimetic activity.

Source: Modified from the 6th Report of the Joint National Committee on Prevention, Detection, Evaluation and Treatment of High Blood Pressure. Arch Intern Med 1997; 157:2413.

HYPERTENSION: INDIVIDUALIZING THERAPY JNC VI

CONSIDERATIONS FOR INDIVIDUALIZING ANTIHYPERTENSIVE DRUG THERAPY

Indication	Drug Therapy
Compelling Indications Unless Contraindicated	
Diabetes mellitus (Type 1) with proteinuria	ACE I
Heart failure	ACE I, diuretics
Isolated systolic hypertension (older patients)	Diuretics (preferred), CA (long-acting DHP)
Myocardial infarction	β-blockers (non-ISA), ACE I (with systolic dysfunction)
May Have Favorable Effects on Comorbid Conditions[a]	
Angina	β-blockers, CA
Atrial tachycardia and fibrillation	β-blockers, CA (non-DHP)
Cyclosporine-induced hypertension (caution with the dose of cyclosporine)	CA
Diabetes mellitus (Types 1 and 2) with proteinuria	
Diabetes mellitus (Type 2)	ACE I (preferred), CA
Dyslipidemia	Low-dose diuretics
Essential tremor	α-Blockers
Heart failure	β-Blockers (non-CS)
Hyperthyroidism	Carvedilol, losartan potassium
Migraine	β-Blockers
Myocardial infarction	β-Blockers (non-CS), CA (non-DHP)
Osteoporosis	Diltiazem hydrochloride, verapamil hydrochloride
Preoperative hypertension	Thiazides
Prostatism (BPH)	β-Blockers
Renal insufficiency (caution in renovascular	α-Blockers
hypertension and creatinine level = 265.2 μmol/L [= 3 mg/dL])	ACE I

HYPERTENSION: IND IVIDUALIZING THERAPY

May Have Unfavorable Effects on Comorbid Conditions[a,b]	
Bronchospastic disease	β-Blockers[c]
Depression	β-Blockers, central α-agonists, reserpine[c]
Diabetes mellitus (types 1 and 2)	β-Blockers, high-dose diuretics
Dyslipidemia	β-Blockers (non-ISA), diuretics (high-dose)
Gout	Diuretics
Second- or third-degree heart block	β-Blockers,[c] CA (non DHP)[c]
Heart failure	β-Blockers (except carvedilol), CA (except amlodipine besylate; felodipine)
	Labetalol hydrochloride, methyldopa[c]
Liver disease	β-Blockers
Peripheral vascular disease	ACE I,[c] angiotensin II-receptor blockers[c]
Pregnancy	Potassium-sparing agents
Renal insufficiency	ACE I, angiotensin II-receptor blockers
Renovascular disease	

ACE I = angiotensin-converting enzyme inhibitors; BPH = benign prostatic hyperplasia; CA = calcium antagonists; DHP = dihydropyridine; ISA = intrinsic sympathomimetic activity; MI = myocardial infarction; non-CS = noncardioselective.

[a]Conditions and drugs are listed in alphabetical order.

[b]These drugs may be used with special monitoring unless contraindicated.

[c]Contraindicated.

Source: Adapted from the 6th Report of the Joint National Committee on Prevention, Detection, Evaluation & Treatment of High Blood Pressure. Arch Intern Med 1997; 157:2413.

ADULT ACUTE LOW BACK PAIN: ALGORITHM 1. INITIAL EVALUATION
Sources: Agency for Healthcare Research and Quality; American Academy of Family Practitioners; American College of Radiology

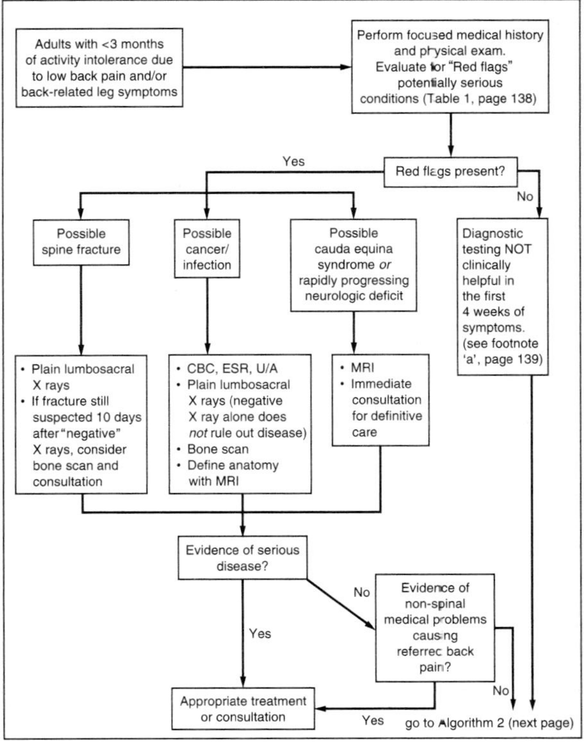

ADULT ACUTE LOW BACK PAIN: ALGORITHM 2. TREATMENT

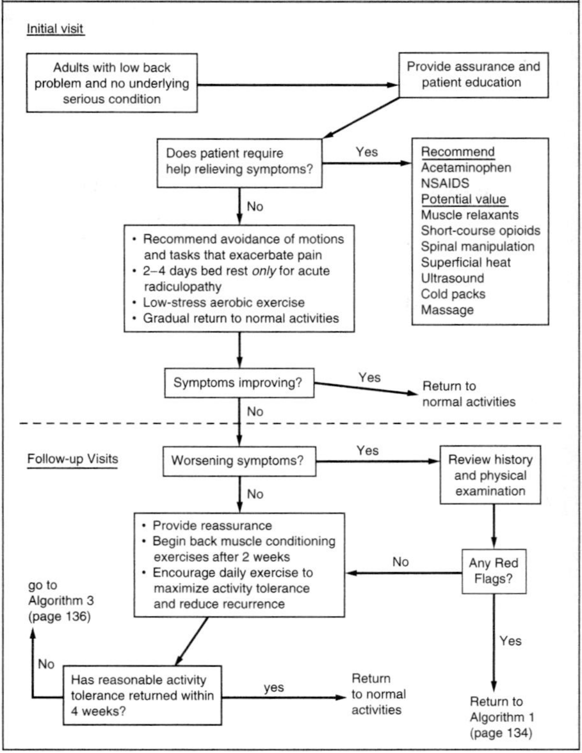

ADULT ACUTE LOW BACK PAIN: ALGORITHM 3. EVALUATION OF SLOW-TO-RECOVER PATIENT (SYMPTOMS >4 WEEKS)

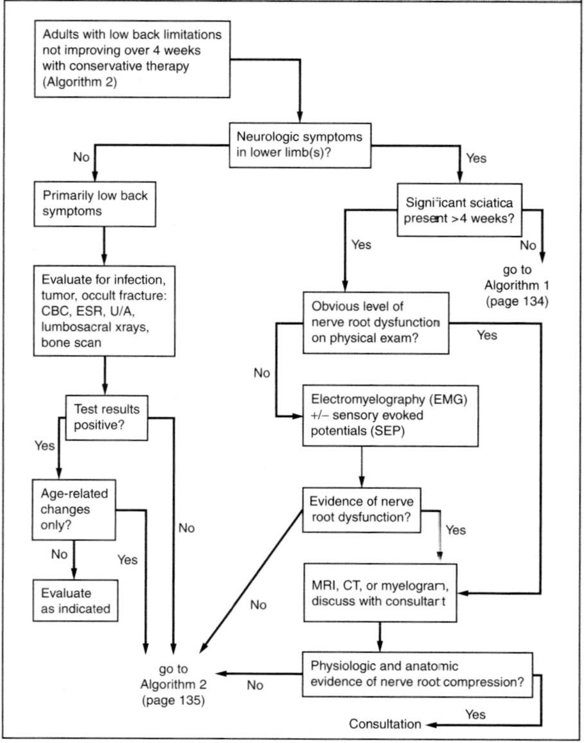

ADULT ACUTE LOW BACK PAIN—PERSISTENT SCIATICA
ALGORITHM 4: SURGICAL CONSIDERATIONS

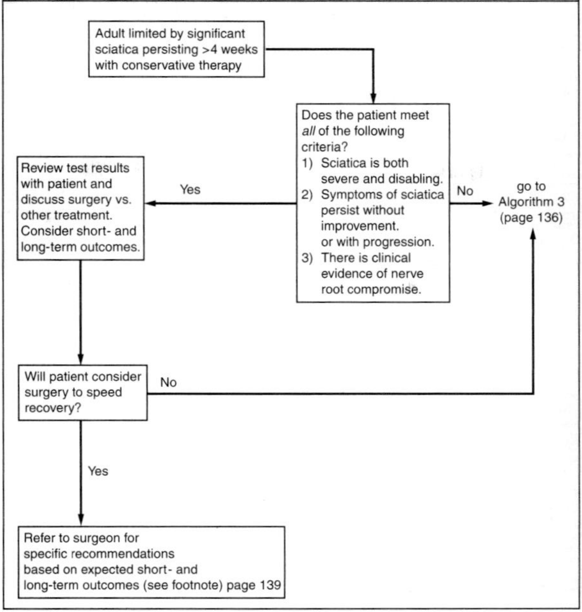

TABLE 1. RED FLAGS FOR POTENTIALLY SERIOUS CONDITIONS

History Features	**Fracture**	**Cancer or Infection**	**Cauda Equina Syndrome**
Major trauma, ie, motor vehicle accident or fall from height	×		
Minor trauma or strenuous lifting (older or osteoporotic patient)	×		
Age > 50 or < 20		×	
History of cancer		×	
Constitutional symptoms (ie, fever, weight loss)		×	
Risk factors for spinal infection (ie, recent bacterial infection, IV drug use, immune suppression)		×	
Pain that worsens when supine		×	
Severe nighttime pain		×	
Saddle anesthesia			×
Recent onset of bladder dysfunction (ie, urinary retention, increased frequency, overflow incontinence)			×
Severe or progressive lower extremity neurologic deficit			×
Physical Examination Features			
Anal sphincter laxity			×
Perianal/perineal sensory loss			×
Major motor weakness: knee extension, foot drop			×

Footnotes for Adult Acute Low Back Pain Algorithms

Footnote to Algorithm 1:[a]

Is has generally been believed that 80–90% of acute low back pain episodes recover spontaneously within 4 weeks. However, more recent studies indicate that there may be a significant percentage of individuals who continue to have pain or functional limitation at 1 year. Recurrences are common, affecting 40% of patients within 6 months. The emerging picture is that of a chronic problem with intermittent exacerbations, rather than an acute disease that can be cured.

Sources:

Deyo RA, Weinstein JM. Low Back Pain. N Engl J Med 2001; 244:363–370.

Cherkin DC, Deyo RA, Street JH, Barlow W. Predicting poor outcomes for back pain seen in primary care using patients' own criteria. Spine 1966; 21:2900–2907.

Croft PR, Macfarlane GJ, Papageorgiou AC, Thomas E, Silman AJ. Outcome of low back pain in general practice: a prospective study. Br Med J 1998; 316:1356–59.

Thomas E, Silman AJ, Croft PR, Papageorgiou AC, Jayson MI V, Macfarlane GJ. Predicting who develops chronic low back pain in primary care: a prospective study. Br Med J 1999; 318:1662–1667.

Footnote to Algorithm 4:

Herniated disk: Surgery for herniated discs is invasive and comprises all types of surgical and injection techniques to remove or reduce the size of herniated intervertebral discs that compress nerve roots. Included are standard discectomy, microscopic discectomy, percutaneous discectomy, and chemonucleolysis.

The therapeutic objective is to relieve pressure on nerve roots and reduce pain and possibly weakness and/or numbness in the lower extremities. Lumbar discectomy may relieve symptoms faster than continued nonsurgical therapy in patients who have severe and disabling leg symptoms and who have not improved after 4–8 weeks of adequate nonsurgical treatment. However, in nonemergent patients, there appears to be little difference in long-term outcomes at 4 and 10 years between discectomy and conservative care.

Spinal stenosis: Elderly patients with spinal stenosis who can adequately function in the activities of daily life can be managed with conservative treatments. Surgery for spinal stenosis should not usually be considered in the first 3 months of symptoms. Decisions on treatment should take into account the patient's lifestyle, preference, other medical problems, and risk of surgery. In one study of patients with severe lumbar spinal stenosis, surgical treatment was associated with greater improvement in patient-reported outcomes than nonsurgical treatment at 4 years (70% vs. 52% reported that their predominant symptom was better). The relative benefit of surgery declined over time but remained superior to nonsurgical treatment. (Atlas SJ, Keller RB, Robson D, Deyo RA, Singer DE. Surgical and nonsurgical management of lumbar spinal stenosis: four-year outcomes from the Maine Lumbar Spine Study. Spine 2000;25:556–62.)

Sources:

Bigos S *et al.* Acute low back problems in adults. Rockville, MD: US Department of Health and Human Services, Public Health Service, Agency for Health Care Policy and Research, 1994. AHCPR Publication no. 95-0642.

Patel AT, Oble AA. Diagnosis and Management of Acute Low Back Pain. Am Fam Physician. 2000;61:1779-86. American College of Radiology. ACR Appropriateness Criteria. www.acr.org. (web site accessed 1/21/01)

OSTEOPOROSIS: EVALUATION & MANAGEMENT

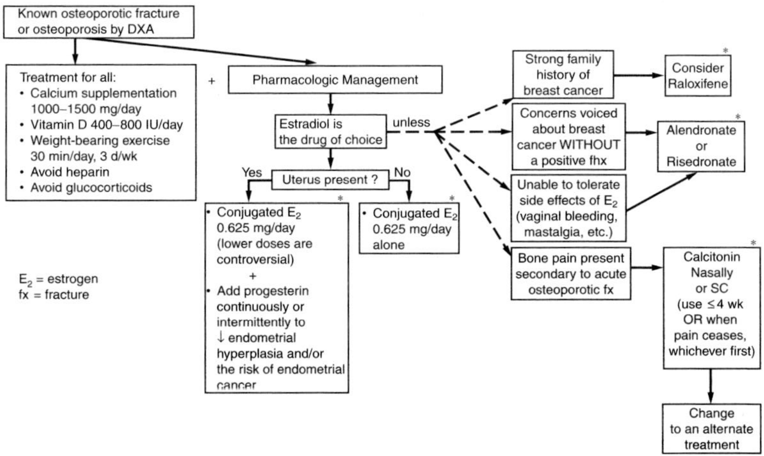

(Adopted from Up To Date "Overview of the Management of Osteoporosis in Women" by H.N. Rosen & M. Rosenblatt)

RISKS AND BENEFITS OF HORMONE REPLACEMENT THERAPY (HRT)[a]

	Risk for Untreated Women (Average)	Risk/Benefit with HRT
Breast Cancer	Lifetime risk 10%	No increased risk with short-term (< 5 years) therapy; risk may be increased with long-term therapy. A recent study suggests that an estrogen-progestin regimen (increased RR = 0.12 per year of treatment) increases breast cancer risk beyond that associated with estrogen alone (increased RR = 0.03 per year of treatment) among women with BMI d 24.4 kg/m^2 (JAMA 2000;283:485)
Coronary Heart Disease (CHD)	46% lifetime probability of developing and 31% risk of dying from CHD After age 60 years, CHD is the primary cause of death for women.	There is 350% less CHD among women who have ever used estrogens, compared with those who have never used them. The only prospective trial of HRT showed no benefit of HRT on CHD events in women with a history of CAD (ie, secondary prevention). (JAMA 1998;280:605)
Endometrial cancer	Lifetime risk 2.6%	With unopposed estrogen, risk is increased 4- to 11-fold. Addition of progestins for at least 10 days per month prevents development of the endometrial hyperplasia associated with unopposed estrogen use.
Osteoporosis	15% lifetime probability of hip fracture (for white women)	Rates of vertebral, wrist, and hip fractures can be reduced by 50–80% after 6–10 years of therapy.

[a]To aid in individualized patient counseling.

Source: Modified, with permission, from Goroll AH, May LA, Mulley AG Jr (eds): Primary Care Medicine: Office Evaluation and Management of the Adult Patient, 3rd ed. Lippincott, 1995. Rosenfeld JA (ed): Women's Health in Primary Care. Williams & Wilkins, 1997.

HORMONE REPLACEMENT THERAPY

HRT TREATMENT REGIMENS FOR WOMEN WITH INTACT UTERI[a]

HRT	Days of Month	Comments
Estrogen Progestin None	1–25 14–25 26–30	97% have withdrawal bleeding until at least age 60 years; after age 65 only 60% continue to bleed.
Estrogen Progestin	1–30 14–25	Avoids estrogen deficiency symptoms.
Estrogen Progestin	1–30 1–30	Avoids cyclic bleeding. During the first 46 months, 35% experience unpredictable spotting and bleeding; by 6 months, 60–65% are amenorrheic.
Estrogen Progestin	1–25 1–25	May provide greater endometrial protection because stopping progestin allows endometrial shedding. Less breakthrough bleeding after the first month than with continuous combined therapy; 75% are amenorrheic by 4 months.

[a]For women without a uterus, progestin is not needed.

Source: Modified, with permission, from Goroll AH, May LA, Mulley AG Jr (eds): Primary Care Medicine: Office Evaluation and Management of the Adult Patient, 3rd ed. Lippincott, 1995. Rosenfeld JA (ed): Women's Health in Primary Care. Williams & Wilkins, 1997.

HORMONE REPLACEMENT THERAPY

HRT: MANAGEMENT OF SYMPTOMS AND SIDE EFFECTS

Symptom/Side Effect	Suggested Intervention
Abdominal bloating	Try lower dose or different progestin. Try hydrochlorothiazide during progestin therapy.
Bleeding on unopposed estrogen or irregular bleeding on combination therapy	Endometerial biopsy
Breakthrough bleeding on combination therapy	Increase progestin dose at 3-month intervals.
Breast tenderness	Lower estrogen dose. Try a different progestin. Consider use of hydrochlorothiazide. Avoid caffeine. Try vitamin E. Evaluate if condition persists.
Decreased libido	Try androgen-estrogen combination.
Migraine headaches	Try transdermal patch. Stop HRT if headaches continue.
Nausea	Often decreases with time. Take medication with food or at bedtime. Try lower doses or transdermal patches.
Persistent menopausal symptoms	Increase estrogen dose or try different estrogen or different delivery system.
Urogenital atrophy	Use topical estrogen. Initiate with daily administration for 34 weeks, then decrease to twice weekly.

Source: Modified from Goroll AH, May LA, Mulley AG Jr (eds): Primary Care Medicine: Office Evaluation and Management of the Adult Patient, 3rd ed. Lippincott, 1995. Rosenfeld JA (ed): Women's Health in Primary Care. Williams & Wilkins, 1997.

APPROACH TO ACUTE COUGH ILLNESS IN ADULTS
Source: Centers for Disease Control and Prevention

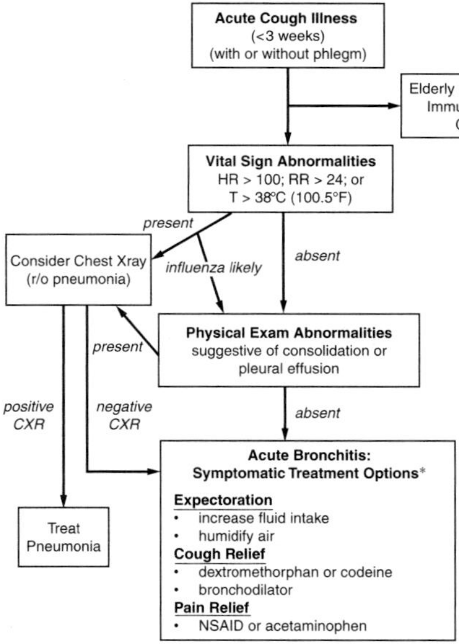

† Pneumonia in the elderly, as well as those with comorbidity, often presents atypically. Evaluation should be individualized.

* If duration of illness is >2 weeks, consider pertussis. PCR or culture testing for pertussis is done to confirm the diagnosis and indicate the need for public health follow-up to prevent illness among contacts, especially infants. Antibiotic therapy can decrease shedding, but has no effect on symptoms during the paroxysmal phase (≥10 days after illness onset). Treat with erythromycin x 14 days pending results.

Adapted from: Centers for Disease Control and Prevention; Ann Intern Med 2001; 134:521

APPROACH TO ACUTE SORE THROAT IN ADULTS
Source: Centers for Disease Control and Prevention

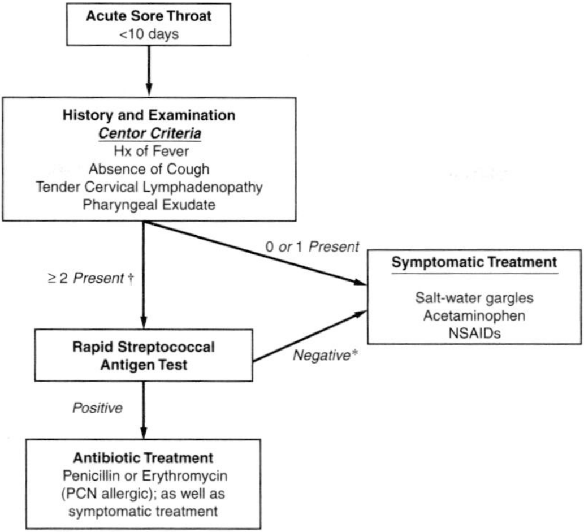

† Acceptable alternatives to these strategies include: 1) test and treat patients with 2 or 3 Centor criteria present, and empirically treat with antibiotics (do not test) patients with 4 Centor criteria; or 2) do not test any patients, and empirically treat with antibiotics patients with 3 or 4 Centor criteria present.

* Do not recommend culture-confirmation of negative rapid antigen tests in adults when the sensitivity of the rapid antigen test exceeds 80%.

These principles apply to immunocompetent adults without complicated comorbidities such as chronic lung or heart disease, history of rheumatic fever, or during known group A streptococcal outbreaks. They also are not intended to apply during a known epidemic of acute rheumatic fever or streptococcal pharyngitis, or for non-industrialized countries where the endemic rate of acute rheumatic fever is much higher than it is in the US.

Adapted from: Centers for Disease Control and Prevention; Ann Intern Med 2001; 134:509

APPROACH TO ACUTE NASAL AND SINUS CONGESTION IN ADULTS
Source: Centers for Disease Control and Prevention

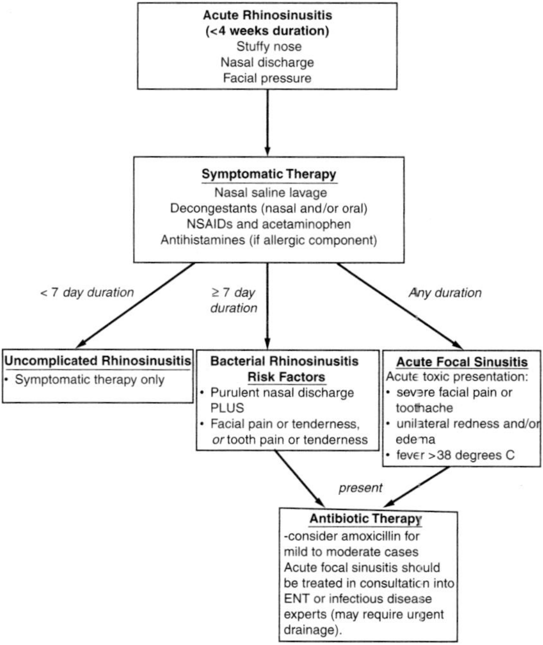

The above principles apply to the diagnosis and treatment of acute maxillary and ethmoid rhinosinusitis in non-immunocompromised adults.

Adapted from: Centers for Disease Control and Prevention; Ann Intern Med 2001;134:498

UTI IN ADULT WOMEN: DIAGNOSIS AND MANAGEMENT
Source: University of Michigan Health System

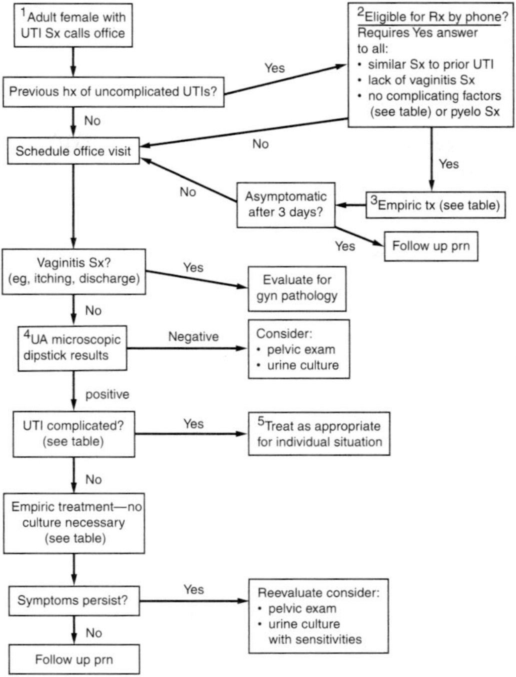

Adapted from: University of Michigan Health System, Urinary Tract Infection guideline, June 1999.

UTI IN ADULT WOMEN ALGORITHM, NOTES AND TABLES

LABORATORY CHARGES AND RELATIVE COSTS

Test	Relative Cost
Urinalysis, dipstick	$
Urinalysis, complete microscopic	$$
Urine culture	$$$

COMPLICATING FACTORS

- Catheter
- Diabetes mellitus
- Immunosuppression
- Nephrolithiasis
- Pregnancy
- Pyelonephritis symptoms
- Recent hospitalization or nursing home residence
- Recurrent UTIs (> 3/year)
- Symptoms for > 7 days
- Urologic structural/functional abnormality

TREATMENT REGIMENS AND RELATIVE COSTS

Treatment Regimen	Relative Cost
First Line	
Trimethoprim/Sulfa DS BID × 3 days	$
Second Line (in preferred order)	
Trimethoprim 100 mg TID × 3 days	$
Ciprofloxacin 100 mg BID × 3 days	$$
Norfloxacin 400 mg BID × 3 days	$$$
Ofloxacin 200 mg BID × 3 days	$$$
Amoxicillin 500 mg TID × 7 days	$$
Nitrofurantoin 100 mg QID × 7 days	$$$$
Nitrofurantoin 100 mg BID × 7 days	$$$

1. The majority of UTIs occur in sexually active women. Risk increases by 3–5 times when diaphragms are used for contraception. Risk also increases slightly with not voiding after sexual intercourse and use of spermicides. Dysuria with either urgency or frequency, in the absence of vaginal symptoms, yields a prior probability of UTI of 70–80%. Generally, UTI symptoms are of abrupt onset (< 3 days).

2. The majority of UTIs in women are uncomplicated and resolve readily with brief courses of antibiotics. Therefore, many women can be assessed and safely managed without an office visit or laboratory examination. A study of a telephone-based clinical practice guideline for managing presumed uncomplicated cystitis among women aged 18–55 years found that guideline implementation significantly decreased the proportion of patients with presumed cystitis who received urinalysis, urine culture, or an initial office visit. The guideline also increased the proportion of women who received a guideline-recommended antibiotic. Adverse outcomes (return office visit, sexually transmitted disease, pyelonephritis within 60 days of initial diagnosis) did not increase as a result of guideline implementation. The study authors concluded that guideline use decreased laboratory utilization and overall costs while maintaining or improving the quality of care for patients who were presumptively treated for acute uncomplicated cystitis. (Saint S, Scholes D, Fihn S, Farrell R, Stamm W. The effectiveness of a clinical practice guideline for the management of presumed uncomplicated urinary tract infection in women. Am J Med 1999; 106:636–641)
3. Acute uncomplicated cystitis in women traditionally has been treated with longer (7–10 day) courses of antibiotics. More recent studies have found shorter courses (3–5 days) of oral antibiotics to be as effective as traditional courses. A review of 28 treatment trials of adult women with uncomplicated cystitis concluded that no benefit was achieved by increasing the length of therapy beyond 5 days. (Norrby SR. Short-term treatment of uncomplicated lower urinary tract infections in women. Rev Infect Dis 1990;12:458–467) The optimal treatment of uncomplicated UTI in patients who are not allergic or sensitive is 3 days of TMP/SMX.
4. <u>Dipstick analysis</u> for leukocyte esterase, an indirect test for the presence for pyuria, is the least expensive and least time-intensive diagnostic test for UTI. It is estimated to have a sensitivity of 75–96% and specificity of 94–98%. Nitrite testing by dipstick is less useful, in large part because it is only positive in the presence of bacteria that produce nitrate reductase, and can be confounded by consumption of ascorbic acid. <u>Microscopic examination</u> of unstained, centrifuged urine by a trained observer under 40 × power has a sensitivity of 82–97% and a specificity of 84–95%. For urine culture, sensitivity varies from 50–95%, depending on the threshold for UTI, and specificity varies from 85–99%. Because of the limited sensitivity of urine culture, and the delay required for results, urine culture is not recommended to diagnose or verify uncomplicated UTI.
5. Unlike women with uncomplicated UTI, care for women with complicating factors includes:
   - <u>Culture:</u> obtain pretreatment culture and sensitivity
   - <u>Treatment:</u> Initiate treatment with trimethoprim/sulfa or quinolone for 7–14 days (quinolones contraindicated in pregnancy)
   - <u>Follow-up UA:</u> obtain follow-up urinalysis to document clearing
   - <u>Possible structural evaluation:</u> Lower threshold for urologic structural evaluation with cysto/IVP.

4
Appendices

SCREENING INSTRUMENTS: ALCOHOL ABUSE

SENSITIVITY AND SPECIFICITY OF SCREENING TESTS FOR PROBLEM DRINKING

Instrument Name	Screening Questions/Scoring	Threshold Score	Sensitivity/Specificity (%)	Source
CAGE[a]	See table below	> 1 > 2 > 3	77/58 53/81 29/92	Am J Psychiatr 1974;131:1121 J Gen Intern Med 1998;13:379
AUDIT	See table below	> 4 > 5 > 6	87/70 77/84 66/90	BMJ 1997;314:420 J Gen Intern Med 1998;13:379

[a]The CAGE may be less applicable to binge drinkers (eg, college students), the elderly, and minority populations.

SCREENING INSTRUMENTS: ALCOHOL ABUSE

SCREENING PROCEDURES FOR PROBLEM DRINKING

1. CAGE screening test[a]

Have you ever felt the need to	**C**ut down on drinking?
Have you ever felt	**A**nnoyed by criticism of your drinking?
Have you ever felt	**G**uilty about your drinking?
Have you ever taken a morning	**E**ye opener?

INTERPRETATION: Two "yes" answers are considered a positive screen. One "yes" answer should arouse a suspicion of alcohol abuse.

2. The alcohol use disorder identification test (AUDIT).[b] (Scores for response categories are given in parentheses. Scores range from 0 to 40, with a cutoff score of ≥ 5 indicating hazardous drinking, harmful drinking, or alcohol dependence.)

1 How often do you have a drink containing alcohol?

(0) Never	(1) Monthly or less	(2) Two to four times a month	(3) Two or three times a week	(4) Four or more times a week

2 How many drinks containing alcohol do you have on a typical day when you are drinking?

(0) 1 or 2	(1) 3 or 4	(2) 5 or 6	(3) 7 to 9	(4) 10 or more

3 How often do you have six or more drinks on one occasion?

(0) Never	(1) Less than monthly	(2) Monthly	(3) Weekly	(4) Daily or almost daily

4 How often during the past year have you found that you were not able to stop drinking once you had started?

(0) Never	(1) Less than monthly	(2) Monthly	(3) Weekly	(4) Daily or almost daily

5 How often during the past year have you failed to do what was normally expected of you because of drinking?

(0) Never	(1) Less than monthly	(2) Monthly	(3) Weekly	(4) Daily or almost daily

continued on next page

SCREENING INSTRUMENTS: ALCOHOL ABUSE

SCREENING PROCEDURES FOR PROBLEM DRINKING (CONTINUED)

6 How often during the past year have you needed a first drink in the morning to get yourself going after a heavy drinking session?

(0) Never (1) Less than monthly (2) Monthly (3) Weekly (4) Daily or almost daily

7 How often during the past year have you had a feeling of guilt or remorse after drinking?

(0) Never (1) Less than monthly (2) Monthly (3) Weekly (4) Daily or almost daily

8 How often during the past year have you been unable to remember what happened the night before because you had been drinking?

(0) Never (1) Less than monthly (2) Monthly (3) Weekly (4) Daily or almost daily

9 Have you or has someone else been injured as a result of your drinking?

(0) No (2) Yes, but not in the past year (4) Yes, during the past year

10 Has a relative or friend or a doctor or other health worker been concerned about your drinking or suggested you cut down?

(0) No (2) Yes, but not in the past year (4) Yes, during the past year

[a]Modified from Mayfield D et al: The CAGE questionnaire: Validation of a new alcoholism screening instrument. Am J Psychiatry 1974;131:1121.

[b]From Piccinelli M et al: Efficacy of the alcohol use disorders identification test as a screening tool for hazardous alcohol intake and related disorders in primary care: A validity study. BMJ 1997;314:420.

SCREENING INSTRUMENTS: COGNITIVE IMPAIRMENT

THE ANNOTATED MINI MENTAL STATE EXAMINATION (AMMSE)

MiniMental LLC

Suspect dementia when score ≤ 24.

NAME OF SUBJECT ____________ Age ________

NAME OF EXAMINER ____________ Years of School Completed ____

Approach the patient with respect and encouragement. Date of Examination ________

Ask: Do you have any trouble with your memory? ☐ Yes ☐ No

May I ask you some questions about your memory? ☐ Yes ☐ No

SCORE ITEM

5 ( ) **TIME ORIENTATION**
Ask:
What is the year ________ (1), season ________ (1),
month of the year ________ (1), date ________ (1),
day of the week ________ (1)?

5 ( ) **PLACE ORIENTATION**
Ask:
Where are we now? What is the state ________ (1), city ________ (1),
part of the city ________ (1), building ________ (1),
floor of the building ________ (1)?

3 ( ) **REGISTRATION OF THREE WORDS**
Say: Listen carefully. I am going to say three words. You say them back after I stop. Ready? Here they are...PONY (wait 1 second), QUARTER (wait 1 second), ORANGE (wait 1 second). What were those words?
________ (1)
________ (1)
________ (1)
Give 1 point for each correct answer, then repeat them until the patient learns all three.

5 ( ) **SERIAL 7s AS A TEST OF ATTENTION AND CALCULATION**
Ask: Subtract 7 from 100 and continue to subtract 7 from each subsequent remainder until I tell you to stop. What is 100 take way 7? ________ (1)
Say:
Keep going. ________ (1), ________ (1),
________ (1), ________ (1),

3 ( ) **RECALL OF THREE WORDS**
Ask:
What were those three words I asked you to remember?
Give one point for each correct answer. ________ (1),
________ (1), ________ (1),

2 ( ) **NAMING**
Ask:
What is this? (show pencil) ________ (1). What is this? (show watch) ________ (1).

For more information or additional copies of this exam, call (617)587-4215

SCREENING INSTRUMENTS: COGNITIVE IMPAIRMENT

MiniMental LLC

1 ( ) **REPETITION**
Say:
Now I am going to ask you to repeat what I say. Ready? No ifs, ands or buts.
Now you say that. ______________________________ (1)

3 ( ) **COMPREHENSION**
Say:
Listen carefully because I am going to ask you to do something.
Take this paper in your left hand (1), fold it in half (1), and put it on the floor. (1)

1 ( ) **READING**
Say:
Please read the following and do what it says, but do not say it aloud. (1)

Close your eyes

1 ( ) **WRITING**
Say:
Please write a sentence. If the patient does not respond, say: Write about the weather. (1)

____

____

1 ( ) **DRAWING**
Say: Please copy this design.

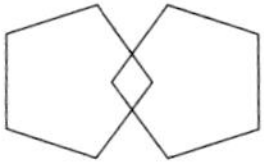

TOTAL SCORE ________ Assess level of consciousness along a continuum

Alert ——— Drowsy ——— Stupor ——— Coma

	YES	NO
Cooperative:	☐	☐
Depressed:	☐	☐
Anxious:	☐	☐
Poor Vision:	☐	☐
Poor Hearing:	☐	☐
Native Language:		
________________		

	YES	NO
Deterioration from previous level of functioning:	☐	☐
Family History of Dementia:	☐	☐
Head Trauma:	☐	☐
Stroke:	☐	☐
Alcohol Abuse:	☐	☐
Thyroid Disease:	☐	☐

FUNCTION BY PROXY
Please record date when patient was last able to perform the following tasks.
Ask caregiver if patient independently handles:

	YES	NO	DATE
Money/Bills:	☐	☐	_____
Medication:	☐	☐	_____
Transportation:	☐	☐	_____
Telephone:	☐	☐	_____

Source: Reproduced, with permission from "MINI-MENTAL STATE." A PRACTICAL METHOD FOR GRADING THE COGNITIVE STATE OF PATIENTS FOR THE CLINICIAN. Journal of Psychiatric Research 1975;12(3):189.

SCREENING INSTRUMENTS: DEPRESSION

SCREENING TESTS FOR DEPRESSION

Instrument Name	Screening Questions/Scoring	Threshold Score	Source
Beck Depression Inventory (Short Form)	See table below	0–4: none or minimal depression 5–7: mild depression 8–15: moderate depression > 15 = severe depression	Postgrad Med 1972;Dec:81
Geriatric Depression Scale	See table below	≥ 15 = depression	J Psychiatr Res 1983;17:37
PRIME-MD© (mood questions)	(1) During the past month, have you often been bothered by feeling down, depressed, or hopeless? (2) During the past month, have you often been bothered by little interest or pleasure in doing things?	"Yes" to either question[a]	JAMA 1994;272:1749 J Gen Intern Med 1997;12:439

[a]Sensitivity 86–96%; specificity 57–75%.
©Pfizer Inc.

SCREENING INSTRUMENTS: DEPRESSION

BECK DEPRESSION INVENTORY, SHORT FORM

Instructions: This is a questionnaire. On the questionnaire are groups of statements. Please read the entire group of statements in each category. Then pick out the one statement in that group that best describes the way you feel today, that is, *right now!* Circle the number beside the statement you have chosen. If several statements in the group seem to apply equally well, circle each one. Sum all numbers to calculate a score.

Be sure to read all the statements in each group before making your choice.

A. Sadness

3 I am so sad or unhappy that I can't stand it.
2 I am blue or sad all the time and I can't snap out of it.
1 I feel sad or blue.
0 I do not feel sad.

B. Pessimism

3 I feel that the future is hopeless and that things cannot improve.
2 I feel I have nothing to look forward to.
1 I feel discouraged about the future.
0 I am not particularly pessimistic or discouraged about the future.

C. Sense of failure

3 I feel I am a complete failure as a person (parent, husband, wife).
2 As I look back on my life, all I can see is a lot of failures.
1 I feel I have failed more than the average person.
0 I do not feel like a failure.

D. Dissatisfaction

3 I am dissatisfied with everything.
2 I don't get satisfaction out of anything anymore.
1 I don't enjoy things the way I used to.
0 I am not particularly dissatisfied.

E. Guilt

3 I feel as though I am very bad or worthless.
2 I feel quite guilty.
1 I feel bad or unworthy a good part of the time.
0 I don't feel particularly guilty.

F. Self-dislike

3 I hate myself.
2 I am disgusted with myself.
1 I am disappointed in myself.
0 I don't feel disappointed in myself.

G. Self-harm

3 I would kill myself if I had the chance.
2 I have definite plans about committing suicide.
1 I feel I would be better off dead.
0 I don't have any thoughts of harming myself.

H. Social withdrawal

3 I have lost all of my interest in other people and don't care about them at all.
2 I have lost most of my interest in other people and have little feeling for them.
1 I am less interested in other people than I used to be.
0 I have not lost interest in other people.

I. Indecisiveness

3 I can't make any decisions at all anymore.
2 I have great difficulty in making decisions.
1 I try to put off making decisions.
0 I make decisions about as well as ever.

J. Self-image change

3 I feel that I am ugly or repulsive-looking.
2 I feel that there are permanent changes in my appearance and they make me look unattractive.
1 I am worried that I am looking old or unattractive.
0 I don't feel that I look any worse than I used to.

SCREENING INSTRUMENTS: DEPRESSION

BECK DEPRESSION INVENTORY, SHORT FORM (CONTINUED)

K. Work difficulty

3 I can't do any work at all.
2 I have to push myself very hard to do anything.
1 It takes extra effort to get started at doing something.
0 I can work about as well as before.

L. Fatigability

3 I get too tired to do anything.
2 I get tired from doing anything.
1 I get tired more easily than I used to.
0 I don't get any more tired than usual.

M. Anorexia

3 I have no appetite at all anymore.
2 My appetite is much worse now.
1 My appetite is not as good as it used to be.
0 My appetite is no worse than usual.

Reproduced, with permission, from Beck AT, Beck RW: Screening depressed patients in family practice: A rapid technic. Postgrad Med 1972;52:81.

GERIATRIC DEPRESSION SCALE

Choose the best answer for how you felt over the past week

1.	Are you basically satisfied with your life?	yes / no
2.	Have you dropped many of your activities and interests?	yes / no
3.	Do you feel that your life is empty?	yes / no
4.	Do you often get bored?	yes / no
5.	Are you hopeful about the future?	yes / no
6.	Are you bothered by thoughts you can't get out of your head?	yes / no
7.	Are you in good spirits most of the time?	yes / no
8.	Are you afraid that something bad is going to happen to you?	yes / no
9.	Do you feel happy most of the time?	yes / no
10.	Do you often feel helpless?	yes / no
11.	Do you often get restless and fidgety?	yes / no
12.	Do you prefer to stay at home, rather than going out and doing new things?	yes / no
13.	Do you frequently worry about the future?	yes / no
14.	Do you feel you have more problems with memory than most?	yes / no
15.	Do you think it is wonderful to be alive now?	yes / no

continued on next page

SCREENING INSTRUMENTS: DEPRESSION

GERIATRIC DEPRESSION SCALE (CONTINUED)

16.	Do you often feel downhearted and blue?	yes / no
17.	Do you feel pretty worthless the way you are now?	yes / no
18.	Do you worry a lot about the past?	yes / no
19.	Do you find life very exciting?	yes / no
20.	Is it hard for you to get started on new projects?	yes / no
21.	Do you feel full of energy?	yes / no
22.	Do you feel that your situation is hopeless?	yes / no
23.	Do you think that most people are better off than you are?	yes / no
24.	Do you frequently get upset over little things?	yes / no
25.	Do you frequently feel like crying?	yes / no
26.	Do you have trouble concentrating?	yes / no
27.	Do you enjoy getting up in the morning?	yes / no
28.	Do you prefer to avoid social gatherings?	yes / no
29.	Is it easy for you to make decisions?	yes / no
30.	Is your mind as clear as it used to be?	yes / no

One point for each response suggestive of depression. (Specifically "no" responses to questions 1, 5, 7, 9, 15, 19, 21, 27, 29, and 30, and "yes" responses to the remaining questions are suggestive of depression.)

A score of ≥ 15 yields a sensitivity of 80% and a specificity of 100%, as a screening test for geriatric depression. (Clin Gerontologist 1982;1:37.)

Reproduced, with permission, from Yesavage JA et al: Development and validation of a geriatric depression screening scale: A preliminary report. J Psychiatr Res 1982–83;17:37.

FUNCTIONAL ASSESSMENT SCREENING IN THE ELDERLY

Target Area	Assessment Procedure	Abnormal Result	Suggested Intervention
Vision	Test each eye with Jaeger card while patient wears corrective lenses (if applicable).	Inability to read greater than 20/40	Refer to ophthalmologist.
Hearing	Whisper a short, easily answered question such as "What is your name?" in each ear while the examiner's face is out of direct view.	Inability to answer question	Examine auditory canals for cerumen and clean if necessary. Repeat test; if still abnormal in either ear, refer for audiometry and possible prosthesis.
Arm	Proximal: "Touch the back of your head with both hands." Distal: "Pick up the spoon."	Inability to do task	Examine the arm fully (muscle, joint, and nerve), paying attention to pain, weakness, limited range of motion. Consider referral for physical therapy.
Leg	Observe the patient after instructing as follows: "Rise from your chair, walk 10 feet, return, and sit down."	Inability to walk or transfer out of chair	Do full neurologic and musculoskeletal evaluation, paying attention to strength, pain, range of motion, balance, and gait. Consider referral for physical therapy.
Continence of urine	Ask, "Do you ever lose your urine and get wet?"	"Yes"	Ascertain frequency and amount. Search for remediable causes, including local irritations, polyuric states, and medications. Consider urologic referral.
Nutrition	Ask, "Without trying, have you lost 10 lbs or more in the last 6 months?" Weigh the patient. Measure height.	"Yes" or weight is below acceptable range for height	Do appropriate medical evaluation.

continued on next page

FUNCTIONAL ASSESSMENT SCREENING IN THE ELDERLY (CONTINUED)			
Target Area	**Assessment Procedure**	**Abnormal Result**	**Suggested Intervention**
Mental status	Instruct as follows: "I am going to name three objects (pencil, truck, book). I will ask you to repeat their names now and then again a few minutes from now."	Inability to recall all three objects after 1 minute	Administer Folstein Mini-Mental Status Examination. If score is less than 24, search for causes of cognitive impairment. Ascertain onset, duration, and fluctuation of overt symptoms. Review medications. Assess consciousness and affect. Do appropriate laboratory tests.
Depression	Ask, "Do you often feel sad or depressed?" or "How are your spirits?"	"Yes" or "Not very good, I guess"	Administer Geriatric Depression Scale. If positive (score above 15), check for antihypertensive, psychotropic, or other pertinent medications. Consider appropriate pharmacologic or psychiatric treatment.
ADL-IADL[a]	Ask, "Can you get out of bed yourself?" "Can you dress yourself?" "Can you make your own meals?" "Can you do your own shopping?"	"No" to any question	Corroborate responses with patient's appearance; question family members if accuracy is uncertain. Determine reasons for the inability (motivation compared with physical limitation). Institute appropriate medical, social, or environmental interventions.
Home environment	Ask, "Do you have trouble with stairs inside or outside of your home?" Ask about potential hazards inside the home with bathtubs, rugs, or lighting.	"Yes"	Evaluate home safety and institute appropriate countermeasures.

FUNCTIONAL ASSESSMENT SCREENING IN THE ELDERLY (CONTINUED)			
Target Area	**Assessment Procedure**	**Abnormal Result**	**Suggested Intervention**
Social support	Ask, "Who would be able to help you in case of illness or emergency?"	. . .	List identified persons in the medical record. Become familiar with available resources for the elderly in the community.

[a]Activities of daily-living-instrumental activities of daily living.

Source: Modified from Lachs MS et al: A simple procedure for screening for functional disability in elderly patients. Ann Intern Med 1990;112:699.

95TH PERCENTILE OF BLOOD PRESSURE FOR BOYS AND GIRLS: BOYS														
	Systolic BP (mm Hg) by percentile of height							Diastolic BP (mm Hg) by percentile of height						
Age (y)	**5%**	**10%**	**25%**	**50%**	**75%**	**90%**	**95%**	**5%**	**10%**	**25%**	**50%**	**75%**	**90%**	**95%**
3	105	106	107	109	111	112	113	63	63	64	65	66	67	68
4	107	108	109	111	113	114	115	67	68	68	69	70	71	72
5	108	109	111	113	114	116	117	71	71	72	73	74	75	76
6	109	110	112	114	116	117	118	74	75	75	76	77	78	79
7	110	111	113	115	117	118	119	77	77	78	79	80	81	81
8	112	113	114	116	118	119	120	79	79	80	81	82	83	83
9	113	114	116	118	119	121	122	80	81	81	82	83	84	85
10	115	116	117	119	121	123	123	81	82	83	83	84	85	86
11	117	118	119	121	123	125	125	82	82	83	84	85	86	87
12	119	120	122	124	125	127	128	83	83	84	85	86	87	87
13	121	122	124	126	128	129	130	83	83	84	85	86	87	88
14	124	125	127	129	131	132	133	83	84	85	86	87	87	88
15	127	128	130	132	133	135	136	84	85	86	86	87	88	89
16	130	131	133	134	136	138	138	86	86	87	88	89	90	90
17	132	133	135	137	139	140	141	88	88	89	90	91	92	93

95TH PERCENTILE OF BLOOD PRESSURE FOR BOYS AND GIRLS: GIRLS

	Systolic BP (mm Hg) by percentile of height							Diastolic BP (mm Hg) by percentile of height						
Age (y)	5%	10%	25%	50%	75%	90%	95%	5%	10%	25%	50%	75%	90%	95%
3	104	104	106	107	108	109	110	65	65	66	66	67	68	68
4	105	106	107	108	109	111	111	68	68	69	69	70	71	71
5	107	107	108	110	111	112	113	71	71	71	72	73	74	74
6	108	109	110	111	113	114	114	73	73	74	74	75	76	76
7	110	111	112	113	114	115	116	75	75	75	76	77	78	78
8	112	113	114	115	116	117	118	76	77	77	78	79	79	80
9	114	115	116	117	118	119	120	78	78	79	79	80	81	81
10	116	117	118	119	120	122	122	79	79	80	81	81	82	83
11	118	119	120	121	122	124	124	81	81	81	82	83	83	84
12	120	121	122	123	125	126	126	82	82	82	83	84	85	85
13	122	123	124	125	126	128	128	83	83	84	84	85	86	86
14	124	125	126	127	128	129	130	84	84	85	85	86	87	87
15	125	126	127	128	130	131	131	85	85	85	86	87	88	88
16	126	127	128	129	130	132	132	85	85	86	87	87	88	88
17	127	127	128	130	131	132	133	85	86	86	87	88	88	89

Source: Adapted, with permission, from Rosner B et al: Blood pressure nomograms for children and adolescents, by height, sex, and age, in the United States. J Pediatr 1993;123:874.

BODY MASS INDEX CONVERSION TABLE			
	BMI 25 kg/m^2	BMI 27 kg/m^2	BMI 30 kg/m^2
Height in inches (cm)	Body weight in pounds (kg)		
58 (147.32)	119 (53.98)	129 (58.51)	143 (64.86)
59 (149.86)	124 (56.25)	133 (60.33)	148 (67.13)
60 (152.40)	128 (58.06)	138 (62.60)	153 (69.40)
61 (154.94)	132 (59.87)	143 (64.86)	158 (71.67)
62 (157.48)	136 (61.69)	147 (66.68)	164 (74.39)
63 (160.02)	141 (63.96)	152 (68.95)	169 (76.66)
64 (162.56)	145 (65.77)	157 (71.22)	174 (78.93)
65 (165.10)	150 (68.04)	162 (73.48)	180 (81.65)
66 (167.64)	155 (70.31)	167 (75.75)	186 (84.37)
67 (170.18)	159 (72.12)	172 (78.02)	191 (86.64)
68 (172.72)	164 (74.39)	177 (80.29)	197 (89.36)
69 (175.26)	169 (76.66)	182 (82.56)	203 (92.08)
70 (177.80)	174 (78.93)	188 (85.28)	207 (93.90)
71 (180.34)	179 (81.19)	193 (87.54)	215 (97.52)
72 (182.88)	184 (83.46)	199 (90.27)	221 (100.25)
73 (185.42)	189 (85.73)	204 (92.53)	227 (102.97)
74 (187.96)	194 (88.00)	210 (95.26)	233 (105.69)
75 (190.50)	200 (90.72)	216 (97.98)	240 (108.86)
76 (193.04)	205 (92.99)	221 (100.25)	246 (111.59)

Metric	Non-metric
Metric conversion formula = weight (kg)/height (m^2) Example of BMI calculation: A person who weighs 78.93 kilograms and is 177 centimeters tall has a BMI of 25: weight (78.93 kg)/height (1.77 m)^2 = 25	**Non-metric conversion formula = [weight (pounds)/height (inches)^2] × 704.5** Example of BMI calculation: A person who weighs 164 pounds and is 68 inches (or 5' 8") tall has a BMI of 25: [weight (164 pounds)/height (68 inches)^2] × 704.5 = 25

Source: Adapted from NHLBI Obesity Guidelines in Adults, 1998

RECOMMENDED CHILDHOOD IMMUNIZATION SCHEDULE (ACIP)

Vaccine	Age[a]										
	Birth	1 mo	2 mo	4 mo	6 mo	12 mo	15 mo	18 mo	4–6 y	11–12 y	14–18 y
HBV[b]	Hep B										
		Hep B			Hep B					Hep B[c]	
DTaP[d]			DTaP	DTaP	DTaP		DTaP[d]		DTaP	Td	
HiB[e]			Hib	Hib	Hib	Hib					
Inactivated polio virus[f]			IPV	IPV	IPV				IPV		
Pneumococcal conjugate[g]			PCV	PCV	PCV		PCV				
MMR[h]						MMR			MMR	MMR[c]	
Varicella[i]						Var				Var[c]	
HAV									Age ≥ 2 years, high risk[j]		
Influenza					For high risk[k]						

Range of acceptable ages for vaccination. Any dose not given at the recommended age should be given as a "catch-up" immunization at any subsequent visit when indicated and feasible.

[a]This schedule indicates the recommended ages for routine administration of currently licensed childhood vaccines, as of 11/1/00. Additional vaccines may be licensed and recommended during the year. Licensed combination vaccines may be used whenever any components of the combination are indicated and its other components are not contraindicated. Providers should consult the manufacturers' package inserts for detailed recommendations.

[b]*Infants of HBsAg-negative mothers:* Should receive the 1st dose of Hep B vaccine by age 2 months. The 2nd dose should be given at least 1 month after the first. The 3rd dose should be administered at least 4 months after the first dose and at least 2 months after the second dose, but not before age 6 months. *Infants of HBsAg-positive mothers:* should receive hepatitis B vaccine and 0.5 mL hepatitis B immune globulin (HBIG) within 12 hours of birth at separate sites. The 2nd dose is recommended at 1–2 months of age, and the 3rd dose at age 6 months. *Infants for whom maternal HBsAg status is unknown:* should receive hepatitis B vaccine within 12 hours of birth. Maternal blood should be drawn at the time of delivery to determine maternal HBsAg status: If the HbsAg is positive, the infant should receive hepatitis B immune globulin as soon as possible (no later than age 1 week). All children and adolescents (through age 18 years) who have not been vaccinated against hepatitis B may begin the series during any visit. Special efforts should be made to vaccinate children who were born in or whose parents were born in areas of the world where HBV infection is moderately or highly endemic.

[c]Vaccines to be assessed and administered if necessary.

[d]The fourth dose of DTaP (diphtheria and tetanus toxoids and acellular pertussis vaccine) may be administered as early as age 12 months, provided 6 months have elapsed since the third dose, particularly if the child is unlikely to return at ages 15–18 months. Td (tetanus and diphtheria toxoids) is recommended at ages 11–12 years if at least 5 years have elapsed since the last dose of DTP, DTaP, or DT. Subsequent routine Td boosters are recommended every 10 years.

[e]Three *Haemophilus influenzae* type b (Hib) conjugate vaccines are licensed for infant use. If PRP-OMP (PedvaxHIB® or ComVax®) is administered at ages 2 and 4 months, a dose at age 6 months is not required. Because clinical studies in infants have demonstrated that using some combination products may induce a lower immune response to the Hib vaccine component, DTaP/Hib combination products should not be used for primary immunization in infants at 2, 4 or 6 months of age, unless FDA-approved for these ages.

[f]An all-IPV schedule is recommended for routine childhood polio vaccination in the United States. All children should receive IPV at 2 months, 4 months, 6–18 months, and 4–6 years of age. Oral polio vaccine (OPV) should be used only in selected circumstances.

[g]The heptavalent conjugate pneumococcal vaccine (PCV) is recommended for all children 2–23 months of age. It also is recommended for certain children 24–59 months of age.

[h]The second dose of MMR is recommended routinely at ages 4–6 years but may be administered during any visit, provided that at least 4 weeks have elapsed since receipt of the first dose and that both doses are administered beginning at or after age 12 months. Those who have not previously received the second dose should complete the schedule no later than the routine visit at ages 11–12 years.

[i]Varicella vaccine is recommended at any visit on or after the first birthday for susceptible children (ie, those who lack a reliable history of chickenpox and who have not been vaccinated). Susceptible persons age ≥ 13 years should receive 2 doses given at least 4 weeks apart.

[j]High risk: persons living in, traveling to, or working in areas where the disease is endemic and periodic outbreaks occur; institutionalized persons; men who have sex with men; injection drug users; military personnel; and certain hospital and laboratory workers. Schedule: 3 doses, with second and third doses given 1 and 6–12 months after the first dose. If patient requires immediate protection against HAV, administer immune globulin simultaneously with the first vaccine dose.

[k]High risk: residents of chronic care facilities and patients with chronic cardiopulmonary disorders, metabolic diseases (including diabetes mellitus), hemoglobinopathies, immunosuppression, and renal dysfunction.

Source: Modified from: Recommended childhood immunization schedule, United States. MMWR Morb Mortal Wkly Rep 2001;50(1):7–10, 19.

RECOMMENDED ADULT IMMUNIZATION SCHEDULE

Vaccine	Age: 18–24 y	25–34 y	35–44 y	45–54 y	55–64 y	65–74 y	≥ 75 y
HBV[a]	If not previously vaccinated	For high risk[b]					
DTP	Td booster every 10 years					Td booster at age 65 years	
HAV	For high risk[c]						
Streptococcus pneumoniae	For high risk[d]					Once	
Influenza	For high risk[e]					Annually (begin at age 50)	
MMR[f]	Women of childbearing age; persons born after 1956 who lack evidence of immunity to measles[f]						
Varicella	Two doses at least 4 weeks apart for susceptible persons[g]						

Shaded bar: Range of acceptable ages for vaccination.

[a]Recommended schedule: initial vaccine, then repeat at 1 and 6 months.

[b]High risk: men who have had sex with men, injection drug users and their sexual partners, patients with a history of sexual activity with multiple partners or history of another sexually transmitted disease, international travelers to countries where HBV is of high or intermediate endemicity, recipients of certain blood products (including hemodialysis patients), and persons in health-related jobs with frequent exposure to blood or blood products. Consider testing antibody response in individuals at very high risk of HBV who are likely to have inadequate antibody response (ie, chronic renal dialysis patients, injection drug users, and those with HIV infection).

[c]High risk: persons living in, traveling to, or working in areas where the disease is endemic and periodic outbreaks occur; institutionalized persons; men who have sex with men; injection drug users; military personnel; and certain hospital and laboratory workers. Schedule: 2 doses, with the second dose 6–12 months after the first. If patient requires immediate protection against HAV, administer immune globulin simultaneously with the first vaccine dose.

[d]High risk: institutionalized persons age ≥ 50 years, chronic cardiac or pulmonary disease, diabetes mellitus, anatomic asplenia, special environments with increased risk of pneumococcal disease (eg, certain Native American and Alaska Native populations), alcoholism, cirrhosis, chronic renal failure, nephrotic syndrome, sickle cell disease, multiple myeloma, metastatic or hematologic malignancy, and acquired or congenital immunodeficiency. Routine revaccination is not recommended but may be appropriate to consider in individuals at highest risk for morbidity and mortality from pneumococcal disease (ie, functional or anatomic asplenia, immunocompromised patients) who were vaccinated > 5 years previously, or if age was < 65 years at the time of primary vaccination.

[e]High risk: residents of chronic care facilities, chronic cardiopulmonary disorders, metabolic diseases (including diabetes mellitus), hemoglobinopathies, immunosuppression, renal dysfunction, and health care providers for and household members of high-risk patients.

[f]Obtain history of vaccination and serology, or offer vaccination. Do not administer rubella vaccine to pregnant women. Women receiving rubella vaccine should not become pregnant for 3 months after vaccination.

[g]Susceptible persons are those who lack a reliable history of chickenpox or were never vaccinated. Consider offering serologic testing to adolescents and adults without a reliable history of infection or immunization.

PROFESSIONAL SOCIETIES & GOVERNMENTAL AGENCIES		
Abbreviation	**Full Name**	**Internet Address**
AACE	American Association of Clinical Endocrinologists	www.aace.com
AAD	American Academy of Dermatology	www.aad.org
AAFP	American Academy of Family Physicians	www.aafp.org
AAO	American Academy of Ophthalmology	www.eyenet.org
AAOHNS	American Academy of Otolaryngology/Head & Neck Surgery	www.entnet.org
AAOS	American Academy of Orthopaedic Surgeons	www.aaos.org
AAP	American Academy of Pediatrics	www.aap.org
ACC	American College of Cardiology	www.acc.org
ACCP	American College of Chest Physicians	www.chestnet.org
ACIP	Advisory Committee on Immunization Practices	wonder.cdc.gov
ACOG	American College of Obstetricians and Gynecologists	www.acog.com
ACP	American College of Physicians	www.acponline.org
ACPM	American College of Preventive Medicine	www.acpm.org
ACR	American College of Radiology	www.acr.org
ACS	American Cancer Society	www.cancer.org
ACSM	American College of Sports Medicine	www.acsm.org
ADA	American Diabetes Association	www.diabetes.org
AGA	American Gastroenterological Association	www.gastro.org
AGS	American Geriatrics Society	www.americangeriatrics.org
AHA	American Heart Association	www.americanheart.org
AHRQ	Agency for Healthcare Research and Quality	www.ahrq.gov
AMA	American Medical Association	www.ama-assn.org
ANA	American Nurses Association	www.nursingworld.org
AOA	American Optometric Association	www.aoanet.org
ASCRS	American Society of Colon and Rectal Surgeons	www.fascrs.org

PROFESSIONAL SOCIETIES & GOVERNMENTAL AGENCIES (CONTINUED)		
Abbreviation	**Full Name**	**Internet Address**
ASCO	American Society of Clinical Oncology	www.asco.org
ASGE	American Society for Gastrointestinal Endoscopy	www.asge.org
ASHA	American Speech-Language-Hearing Association	www.asha.org
ATA	American Thyroid Association	www.thyroid.org
ATS	American Thoracic Society	www.thoracic.org
AUA	American Urological Association	auanet.org
CDC	Centers for Disease Control and Prevention	www.cdc.gov
CTF	Canadian Task Force on the Periodic Health Examination	www.hc-sc.gc.ca
NCI	National Cancer Institute	cancernet.nci.nih.gov
NEI	National Eye Institute	www.nei.nih.gov
GAPS	Guidelines for Adolescent Preventitive Services	
NHLBI	National Heart, Lung, and Blood Institute	www.nhlbi.nih.gov
NIDR	National Institute of Dental and Craniofacial Research	www.nidr.nih.gov
NIHCDC	National Institutes of Health Consensus Development Conference	http://consensus.nih.gov
NOF	National Osteoporosis Foundation	www.nof.org
NTSB	National Transportation Safety Board	www.ntsb.gov
SCF	Skin Cancer Foundation	www.skincancer.org
SGIM	Society for General Internal Medicine	www.sgim.org
USPSTF	United States Preventive Services Task Force	www.ahcpr.gov/clinic/uspsfact.htm

REFERENCES

American Academy of Pediatrics and American College of Obstetricians and Gynecologists: Guidelines for Perinatal Care, 4th ed. American College of Obstetricians and Gynecologists, 1997. (referred to as "AAP and ACOG" in tables)

American College of Obstetricians and Gynecologists: Guidelines for Women's Health Care. American College of Obstetricians and Gynecologists, 1996. (referred to as "ACOG" in tables)

American College of Physicians: Guide for Adult Immunization, 3rd ed. American College of Physicians, 1994.

The Canadian Task Force on the Periodic Health Examination: The Canadian Guide to Clinical Preventive Health Care. Minister of Public Works and Government Services Canada, 1994. (Referred to as "CTF" in tables)

The Clinician's Handbook of Preventive Services, 2nd ed. U.S. Public Health Service, International Medical Publishing, Inc., 1998.

Eddy DM: Common Screening Tests. American College of Physicians, 1991.

Elster AB (editor): American Medical Association. AMA Guidelines for Adolescent Preventive Services (GAPS): Recommendations and Rationale. Williams & Wilkins, 1994. (Referred to as "GAPS" in tables)

Green M (editor): Bright Futures: Guidelines for Health Supervision of Infants, Children, and Adolescents. National Center for Education in Maternal and Child Health, 1994. (Referred to as "Bright Futures" in tables)

U.S. Preventive Services Task Force: Guide to Clinical Preventive Services, 2nd ed. Williams & Wilkins, 1996. (Referred to as "USPSTF" in tables)

Index

H

I